Anatomy and Physiology

Anatomy and Physiology

EVELYN FRANK BURNS, M.Ed., R.T.(R)

Division of Health Sciences
Houston Community College System
Houston, Texas

SERIES EDITOR

STEWART C. BUSHONG, Sc.D., F.A.C.R., F.A.C.M.P.

Professor of Radiologic Science, Department of Radiology, Baylor College of Medicine, Houston, Texas

Illustrations by Holly R. Fischer, MFA
Ann Arbor, Michigan

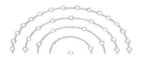

ESSENTIALS OF MEDICAL IMAGING SERIES

McGraw-Hill

Health Professions Division

New York   St. Louis   San Francisco   Auckland   Bogotá   Caracas   Lisbon   London   Madrid
Mexico City   Milan   Montreal   New Delhi   San Juan
Singapore   Sydney   Tokyo   Toronto

McGraw-Hill

A Division of The **McGraw·Hill** *Companies*

ANATOMY AND PHYSIOLOGY

Essentials of Medical Imaging Series

1 2 3 4 5 6 7 8 9 0   DOCDOC   9 9 8

ISBN 0-07-009231-1

This book was set in Berkeley by V&M Graphics.
The editors were John J. Dolan and Peter McCurdy.
The production supervisor was Heather A. Barry.
The text designer was José R. Fonfrias.
The cover designer was Robert Freese.
Malloy Lithographing, Inc. was printer and binder.

This book is printed on acid-free paper.

Visit The McGraw-Hill Health Professions Website at http://www.mghmedical.com

Cataloging-in-Publication data is on file for this title at the Library of Congress.

Dedicated to:

My father, Howard Lindsay Frank,
and the memory of my mother, Martha Evelyn Frank,
for their love and support for my entering a profession that I have always loved.

And to Mary Lou Phillips and the late Robert I. Phillips,
who have served as mentors and always encouraged me
to complete higher level challenges in my career
and for that I will always be grateful.

Contents

Preface

The purpose of this book is to provide a comprehensive review textbook in radiographic anatomy and physiology. The fundamental concepts and anatomy are presented in bulleted fashion to provide a rapid review of basic information.

The illustrations have been provided to use with the text as review material for comprehensive examinations. The format should provide an efficient and thorough review for all levels of students and radiographers. To facilitate the reader's review, terminology lists are provided at the end of each chapter along with a short review test.

The content of this text is not intended to serve as a comprehensive radiographic anatomy and physiology textbook but as a text to be used by students preparing for comprehensive examinations and licensure and certification examinations and as a review of general radiographic anatomy for improvement of positioning.

ACKNOWLEDGMENTS

This manuscript is a culmination of lecture notes and materials developed during my years of teaching students in the Radiography Program at Houston Community College System. I am very thankful to many supporters in helping me complete this project.

To my husband, Barry, I owe a great deal of thanks for his encouragement and assurance that I could complete this project and for his help in keeping the household running as I tried to meet each of the deadlines.

To Teresa Rice, Radiography Program Department Chair and Lynne Davis, Clinical Coordinator, I owe many thanks for their support and willingness to read rough drafts and keep me truly focused on the subject matter. Together, they did an excellent job reviewing the manuscript to make sure the sequencing of information was appropriate.

I have been extremely blessed by the support and encouragement of my Dean (and boss) Dr. Norma Perez, who continues to believe in me and pushes me toward meeting each challenge that comes before me. Thanks again Norma.

A very special thank you is for Holly Fischer, the artist who prepared the illustrations. They speak for themselves.

Preparing this manuscript has been a great experience with the support of the McGraw-Hill Health Professions Division team of John Dolan and Peter McCurdy. Thank you for being so easy to work with and for making this book a success.

EVELYN FRANK BURNS

Introduction to Anatomy and Physiology

TERMINOLOGY

- *Anatomy* is the branch of science that deals with body structure and parts.

- *Physiology* is the study of the function of body parts.

- *Pathology* is the study of disease.

- *Etiology* is the study of the causes of disease.

CHARACTERISTICS OF THE HUMAN ORGANISM

- In order to survive, the human organism must carry out certain processes, processes that cleanse and nourish the body. They include metabolism, removal of waste, response to stimuli, growth, respiration, reproduction for producing new cells as well as for continuation of the human species, digestion, circulation, absorption, and movement.

- The human organism is also required to maintain the internal environment or maintain *homeostasis.*

ORGANIZATION OF THE BODY

- *Cells* are the basic units of the body structure and have specialized functions. *Organelles,* located in the cytoplasm of cells, are small organs that carry out very specialized activities such as the production of molecules of protein, carbohydrates, lipids, and nucleic acids.

- The body is organized into *tissues,* each of which is a group of cells with a common function.

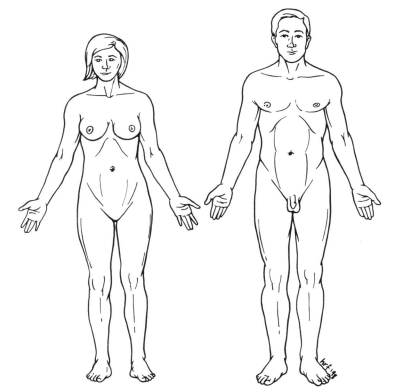

Anterior view human body: Female and male

- Groups of tissues that perform a special function are called *organs*.

- A *system* is a group of organs working in unison to perform specific functions.

- The body is organized by systems.

DIVISIONS OF THE HUMAN ORGANISM

- The human organism consists of an appendicular and an axial skeleton.

- The *appendicular* skeleton includes the arms and legs.

- The *axial* skeleton is made up of the head, neck, and trunk, which has two major cavities called the dorsal and ventral cavities.

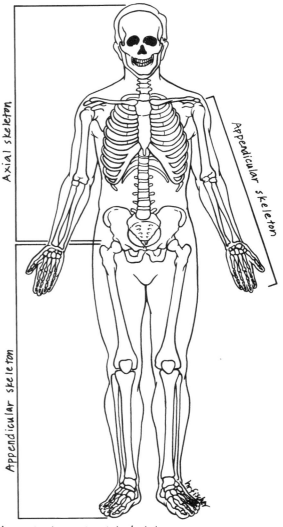

Appendicular and axial skeleton.

- The *dorsal cavity* holds the organs of the cranium (brain) and spinal column (spinal cord and vertebrae).

- The *ventral cavity* has three sections:

1. The *thoracic cavity* contains the lungs, heart and membranous coverings of the heart, mediastinum, thymus, esophagus, and pleural membranes.
2. The *abdominal cavity* contains the peritoneum, liver, gallbladder, pancreas, spleen, stomach, small intestine, most of the large intestine, ureters, and major blood vessels.
3. The *pelvic cavity* contains the distal end of the large intestine, reproductive organs, rectum, and bladder.

BODY PLANES, QUADRANTS, AND REGIONS

- In positioning the human body for examination, radiographers must be familiar with the *body planes, quadrants,* and *regions of the trunk,* and with the *body habitus* (body build or shape), all of which are used to locate specific organs.

- Planes are designated in reference to the anatomical position. The *anatomical position* refers to the position of a person standing erect, raised slightly on the toes, facing forward, and with the arms by the sides with palms facing forward. This position is used to determine what organs lie on the left and right sides of the body.

- The *midsagittal plane* divides the body equally into left and right sections.

- A *sagittal plane* can be on either side of the midsagittal plane and divides the body into left and right sections (not necessarily equal).

- The *coronal plane* divides the body longitudinally and at right angles to the midsagittal plane, resulting in anterior and posterior sections.

- The *transverse plane* divides the body horizontally and at right angles to both the coronal and midsagittal planes.

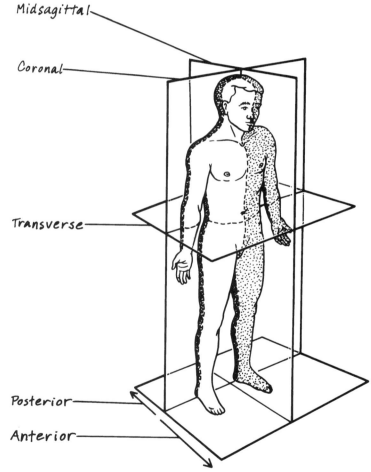

Body in anatomical position demonstrating midsagittal, coronal and transverse planes.

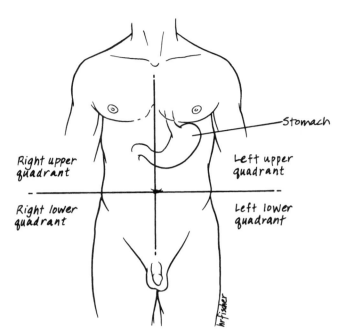

A. The four quadrants of the abdominal cavity.

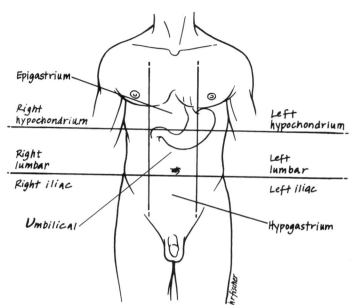

B. The nine regions of the abdominal cavity.

- The trunk of the body is divided into *quadrants:* right upper quadrant, left upper quadrant, right lower quadrant, and left lower quadrant.

- The abdominal cavity is divided into nine *regions:* right and left hypochondriac, right and left lumbar, right and left iliac, epigastric, umbilical, and hypogastric.

BODY BUILD OR HABITUS

- Most people have bodies with a shape, size, general muscle tone, and motility of internal organs that are characteristic of a specific body type or habitus.

- There are four basic *body habitus* types: sthenic, hypersthenic, hyposthenic, and asthenic.

- The *sthenic* type is the most normal or average body shape and represents about 50 percent of the population.

- *Hypersthenic* refers to a large, muscular body with a broad, deep chest and horizontal ribs; the lungs are short, the diaphragm rests high, and the abdomen is long; the gallbladder is high and lies more laterally and horizontally; the stomach is also high in the abdomen.

- *Asthenic* represents an extremely slender body type with a narrow, shallow thoracic cavity; the lungs are longer than in other body types, and therefore the diaphragm is lower; there is a short abdominal cavity with the stomach and gallbladder low in the abdomen and near the midsagittal plane; the large intestine is also lower in the abdomen.

- The *hyposthenic* body type combines characteristics of both the sthenic and asthenic types, generally being a slight modification of the asthenic.

BODY SYSTEMS

- To carry out the specialized activities required for survival of the organism, the body utilizes many systems that perform specific functions.

- The *integumentary system* covers the body, serving to protect the organism in addition to functioning in secretion and absorption.

- The *skeletal* and *muscular systems* work together to provide support for body organs and in the movement of body parts.

- The *nervous* and *endocrine systems* have very complex functions and play an important role in coordinating and integrating other body systems.

- The *digestive* system is responsible for processing and absorbing food nutrients in order to nourish the body's cells.

- The *respiratory system* serves in processing and transportation of molecules and aids in the intake of oxygen which is needed for metabolism.

- The *circulatory system* transports materials from one part of the body to another.

- The *lymphatic system* also functions in processing and transportation of tissue substances.

- The *urinary system* functions include transportation and elimination of waste materials.

- The *reproductive system* plays the vital role of producing new cells and is responsible for continuation of the human species.

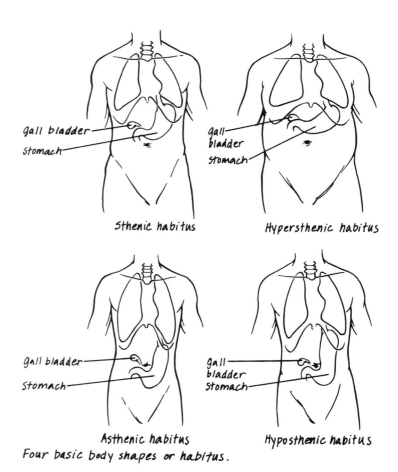

Four basic body shapes or habitus.

RADIOGRAPHIC ANATOMIC TERMINOLOGY

- The following is a list of anatomic terms important to radiographers:

  Anterior toward the front or in front of another organ

  Caudal toward the feet

  Cephalic toward the head

  Distal away from the origin or away from the middle

  Lateral toward the side or at the side

  Medial toward the middle or nearest the middle

  Posterior toward the back or in back of another organ

  Proximal toward the origin or the middle.

Chapter 1 Practice Questions

1. **A group of organs that work together to perform a specific function is called a (an)**

   a. organelle.

   b. cell.

   c. tissue.

   d. system.

2. **The most basic functional unit of the body is the**

   a. organelle.

   b. cell.

   c. organ.

   d. tissue.

3. **Maintaining the internal environment of the body is a major function of organ systems working together. This condition is called**

   a. digestion.

   b. hemostasis.

   c. homeostasis.

   d. respiration.

4. **The axial skeleton is composed of which of the following sets of structures?**

   a. lungs, shoulder girdle, liver, and upper extremities

   b. upper arms, legs, pelvic girdle, and shoulder girdle

   c. head, neck, upper torso, arms, and shoulder girdle

   d. head, neck, dorsal cavity, and ventral cavity

5. **The plane that divides the body into equal left and right parts is the**

   a. midsagittal plane.

   b. sagittal plane.

   c. coronal plane.

   d. transverse plane.

6. The plane that divides the body longitudinally into anterior and posterior sections is the

    a. midsagittal plane.
    b. sagittal plane.
    c. coronal plane.
    d. transverse plane.

7. Which of the following is the most superior and middle region of the abdominal cavity?

    a. the umbilical region
    b. the hypogastric region
    c. the right and left hypochondriac regions
    d. the epigastric region

8. The most normal or average body build or shape is the

    a. sthenic.
    b. asthenic.
    c. hypersthenic.
    d. hyposthenic.

9. Which of the following body systems covers the body and functions in secretion and absorption?

    a. skeletal system
    b. muscular system
    c. integumentary system
    d. circulatory system

10. Which of the following systems functions to coordinate and integrate the activities of other body systems?

    a. nervous system
    b. respiratory system
    c. circulatory system
    d. reproductive system

Match each of the following organs with the correct cavity in which it is located.

11. Heart and lungs _____

12. Spinal cord _____

13. Reproductive organs _____

14. Esophagus _____

15. Peritoneum _____

    a. dorsal
    b. abdominal
    c. thoracic
    d. pelvic

General Organization and Functions of Cells and Tissue

THE CELL

- The basic *building blocks* of the human organism are cells, and there are about 75 trillion cells in the adult body.

- Cells vary in shape and function. The shape is usually related to the function of the cell.

- The structure of a cell consists of a *nucleus* enclosed by a *nuclear membrane*. Outside the nuclear membrane is *cytoplasm* enclosed by a *cell membrane*.

- The cytoplasm consists of a network of membranes and tiny organs called *organelles*. Each organelle performs a specific function related to metabolism.

- The cell membrane can be highly specialized, allowing certain substances to enter and leave the cell.

- Osmosis and diffusion are processes that facilitate the movement of certain substances, such as glucose and water, through the cell membrane. *Osmosis* is the movement of water through a semipermeable membrane from an area of higher concentration to an area of lower concentration until equilibrium is reached. *Diffusion* is the movement of ions or molecules from an area of higher concentration to an area of lower concentration until equilibrium is reached.

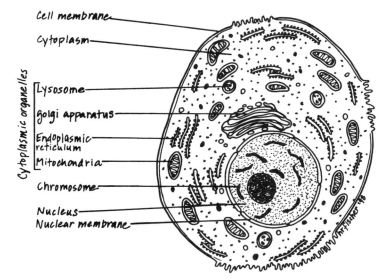

Cell membrane
Cytoplasm
Cytoplasmic organelles
Lysosome
Golgi apparatus
Endoplasmic reticulum
Mitochondria
Chromosome
Nucleus
Nuclear membrane

Structures of typical human cell.

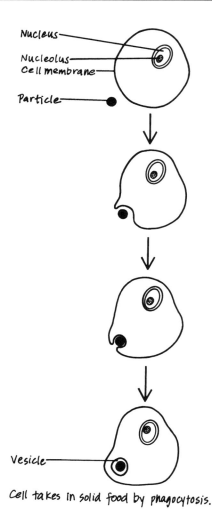

Nucleus
Nucleolus
Cell membrane
Particle

Vesicle

Cell takes in solid food by phagocytosis.

- Cells are able to take in solid particles by a process called *phagocytosis* or "cell eating."

- These processes (osmosis, diffusion, and phagocytosis) allow movement of substances across the cell membranes and contribute to homeostasis which maintains the stability of the cell's internal environment.

- The *nucleus* directs the cell's activities and is the source of the DNA molecules that serve as the cell's blueprint.

- The *shape* of a cell may be directly related to its function. The shape varies, as in the case of a *nerve cell* which may have a main body with long extensions that serve in transmitting messages via nerve impulses to all parts of the body.

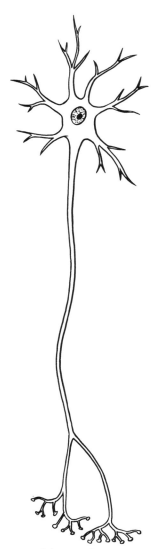

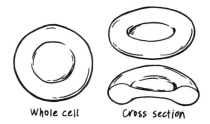

Whole cell   Cross section

A. Red blood cell (erythrocyte).   **B. Nerve cell (neuron).**

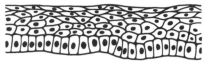

Stratified squamous epithelium

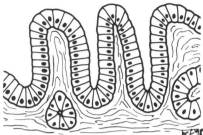

Simple columnar epithelium

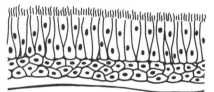

Pseudostratified ciliated columnar epithelium

Examples of multiple types of epithelial tissue.

- *Epithelial cells*, for example, are flat and scale-like, and these cells serve to cover other cells.

- *Muscle cells* are shaped like long fibers and are joined together to facilitate muscle contraction and movement of body parts.

- Most cells grow and then divide by *mitosis*, producing a daughter cell with the same DNA blueprint. Cells continuously produce new cells.

- *Hyperplasia* is the uncontrolled reproduction of cells.

- *Anaplasia* is a process in which the cell structure is abnormal, which possibly prevents it from functioning properly.

- *Metastasis* is the spreading of abnormal cells, such as cancer cells, to other parts of the body.

BODY TISSUE

- Groups of cells that perform a similar function are called *tissue*.

- There are four basic types of tissue in the body: epithelial, connective, muscle, and nerve.

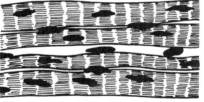

Striated muscle tissue found in skeletal muscle

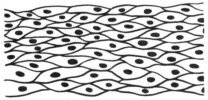

Smooth muscle found in alimentary canal

Examples of muscle tissue.

- *Epithelial tissue* covers the body inside and out. This type of tissue can be found in organs and in glands. Skin, for example, is composed of layers of epithelial tissue.

- Most epithelial cells lack blood vessels and must depend on the cells directly below them for nourishment.

- Epithelial tissue consists of tightly packed cells with functions that include secretion, excretion, and absorption. Epithelial tissue can also act as receptors.

- Epithelial cells divide continuously; for example, old cells on the skin are sloughed off as new cells rise to the surface.

Connective Tissue

- *Connective tissue* is found throughout the body and performs *multiple functions*. These functions include holding structures together such as muscle and bone. Bones are a type of connective tissue that provide a framework and support for the body.

- Connective tissue functions to produce blood cells and to protect against infection; it can also repair damaged cells.

- Additional functions include acting as general space fillers and storing fat.

- Types of connective tissue are *adipose* or *fatty tissue, fibrous tissue, bone,* and *cartilage.*

- The cell types found in connective tissue are fibroblasts and macrophages, as well as mast cells and other cells.

- *Macrophages* are infection fighters and scavengers and eat foreign particles in tissue.

- *Mast cells* are a type of connective tissue located near blood cells that produce *heparin* which helps form blood clots. Mast cells also contain *histamine* which promotes reactions associated with inflammation and allergies.

- *Bone* is the most rigid type of connective tissue. The rigidity or hardness of bone is a result of numerous deposits of mineral salts.

- *Blood* is a type of connective tissue and is made up of cells suspended in blood plasma.

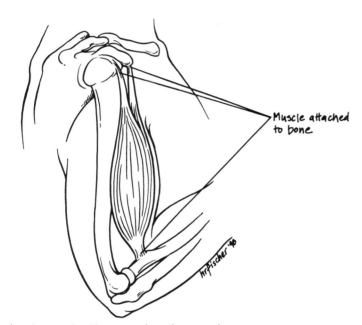

Muscle attached to bone

Joints demonstrating muscle attachment.

- *Muscles* are specialized connective tissue named separately and specialize in contraction involved in movement of the skeleton and in peristaltic movement associated with transportation of substances through vessels and tubes.

- The *heart* is specialized muscle that functions in pumping blood throughout the body.

- The final type of connective tissue is nerve tissue. *Nerve tissue* is found in the brain, spinal cord, and peripheral nerves and provides a pathway for nerve impulses to travel from one point in the body to another.

- Nerve tissue responds to changes in the environment and transmits impulses required for the coordination and regulation of body activities.

PATHOPHYSIOLOGIC TERMINOLOGY ASSOCIATED WITH CELLS AND TISSUE

Adenocarcinoma a malignant tumor of glandular tissue

Carcinoma a malignant tumor

Basal cell carcinoma a malignant tumor of the epithelium

Cellulitis a bacterial infection involving subcutaneous tissue

Chondrosarcoma a malignant tumor of cartilaginous tissue

Edema swelling of tissue usually associated with the accumulation of fluid

Infection invasion of tissue by pathogenic microorganisms which may be bacterial or viral

Inflammation swelling of tissue accompanied by pain, redness, and heat and caused by injury to the tissue; some inflammations may become infections

Melanoma a malignant tumor found in the pigment cells (melanocytes) of the skin

Neoplasm excessive development of tissue during cell division; also called a tumor

Malignant neoplasm a cancerous tumor whose cells may spread to another part of the body

Sarcoma a malignant tumor of connective tissue.

Chapter 2 Practice Questions

1. The small organs that are located within the cytoplasm and function in specific roles during cellular metabolism are called the
   a. nuclei.
   b. nuclear membranes.
   c. organelles.
   d. cell membranes.

2. The process in which ions or molecules move from an area of higher concentration to an area of lower concentration to reach equilibrium is called
   a. osmosis.
   b. diffusion.
   c. homeostasis.
   d. phagocytosis.

3. The "director" of the activities of the cell and the source of the cell's DNA is the
   a. nucleus.
   b. **cytoplasm.**
   c. organelles.
   d. cell membrane.

4. The uncontrolled production of cells is known as
   a. anaplasia.
   b. mitosis.
   c. metastasis.
   d. hyperplasia.

5. The type of tissue that covers most of the body inside and out is called
   a. epithelial tissue.
   b. connective tissue.
   c. muscle tissue.
   d. nerve tissue.

6. Bone and cartilage are considered to be which type of body tissue?
   a. epithelial tissue
   b. connective tissue
   c. muscle tissue
   d. nerve tissue

7. Which of the following cell types found in connective tissue functions in the production of heparin to help form blood clots?
   a. phagocytes
   b. macrophages
   c. fibroblasts
   d. mast cells

8. Blood is considered to be which type of body tissue?
    a. epithelial tissue
    b. connective tissue
    c. muscle tissue
    d. nerve tissue

9. The invasion of tissue by pathogenic microorganisms is called
    a. infection.
    b. inflammation.
    c. edema.
    d. neoplasm.

10. Swollen tissue accompanied by pain, redness, and heat and caused by trauma is called
    a. infection.
    b. inflammation.
    c. edema.
    d. neoplasm.

The Skeleton: Part One Bone Structure and Physiology

BONE STRUCTURE

- The skeleton is the frame for the body, providing *support* for organs and systems.

- Approximately 206 bones make up the human skeleton.

- The skeleton is a composite of tissue types which includes bone, cartilage, blood, nerves, and fibrous connective tissue.

- The skeleton is composed of bones with multiple shapes, including long, short, flat, and irregular bones. Examples are the femur and humerus which are long bones, carpal and tarsal bones which are short bones, the sternum and scapula which are flat bones, and vertebrae which are irregularly shaped bones.

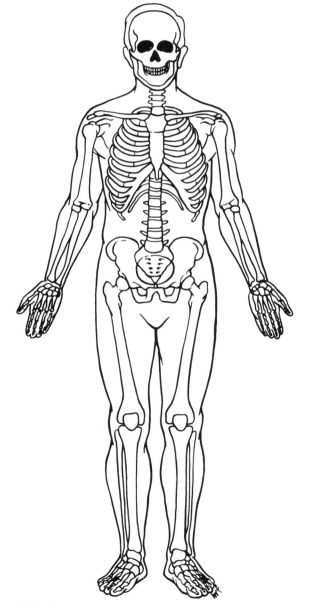

The human skeleton.

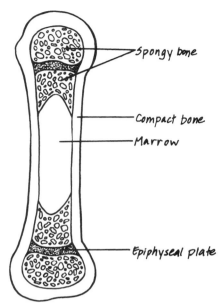

Spongy bone

Compact bone

Marrow

Epiphyseal plate

Developing long bone with epiphyseal disks;
location of compact and spongy bone.

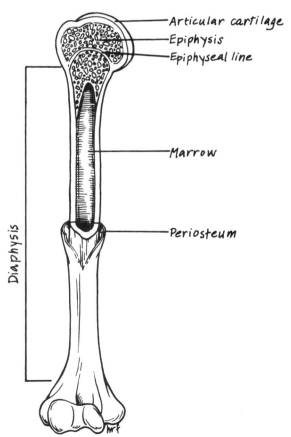

Articular cartilage
Epiphysis
Epiphyseal line

Diaphysis

Marrow

Periosteum

Long bone demonstrating epiphysis, diaphysis,
periosteum, articular cartilage and marrow cavity.

- The long bones, such as the femur, humerus, tibia, and fibula, have an expanded portion at each end called the *epiphysis*. The epiphyseal portion, or the end, of a long bone usually articulates with other bone(s) to create a joint.

- Between the proximal and distal epiphyses is the long portion of the bone called the *diaphysis*.

- The wall of the diaphysis is composed of hard or compact bone which provides a strong, rigid support for weight-bearing long bones.

- The ends or epiphyses of long bones are composed largely of spongelike bone known as *cancellous* bone.

- Cancellous bone is surrounded by a thin layer of compact bone.

- Most short, flat, and irregular bones are composed mainly of cancellous bone covered with a layer of *compact bone*.

- There is radiographic significance in the development of long bones. In children and teenagers a band of cartilage that is not fully calcified (the epiphyseal disk or plate) is seen on radiographs between the diaphysis and the epiphyses. Images must provide radiologists with the capability to differentiate between normal bone growth and a damaged epiphyseal disk. A normal growth pattern may look like a fracture, or vice versa. If damaged, an epiphyseal disk can ossify too early and affect growth to normal bone size.

- The articular surface of bones is covered with a layer of *articular cartilage*.

- The bones are covered entirely, except for the articular surface, with a thin, fibrous membrane called the *periosteum*.

- Bone is formed by cells called *osteoblasts*. Bone development originates in the embryo with fibrous membranes and cartilage forming ossification centers containing osteoblasts. Bone development continues until about 22 to 24 years of age.

- A mature bone cell is called an *osteocyte*. Osteocytes function in the maintenance of bone development and in the repair of bone tissue.

- An *oosteoclast* is a destructive bone cell which plays an important role in the development of long bones of the skeleton and in the removal of tissue during the repair of damaged bone.

FUNCTIONS OF THE SKELETON

- The skeleton serves to support and protect the organs of the body.

- The skull protects the brain, and the vertebrae protect the spinal cord.

- The bony thorax protects the lungs and heart.

- The pelvis is a basin that holds and protects lower abdominal structures and the reproductive organs.

- The skeletal system cooperates with the muscular system to produce movement of body parts.

- Bone marrow, located in the medulla (an inner cavity of long bones), functions to produce red blood cells, white blood cells, and platelets and serves as storage for fat tissue.

- Bones store mineral salts including calcium phosphate. Calcium is a mineral essential for metabolism.

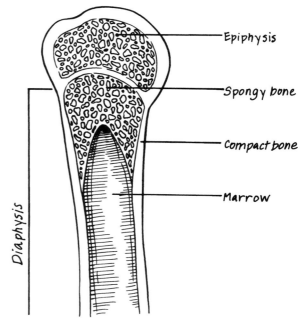

Bone marrow located in diaphyseal section of bone.

DIVISIONS OF THE SKELETON

- The skeleton is divided into an appendicular and an axial skeleton.

Appendicular Skeleton

- The *appendicular skeleton* includes the arms, the legs, and the joints that anchor the bones of the upper and lower limbs, the shoulder and pelvic girdles, respectively.

- The bones of the appendicular skeleton are

   The *upper limbs,* including the humerus, radius, ulna, carpals, metacarpals, and phalanges
   The *shoulder girdle,* including the scapula and clavicle
   The *lower limbs,* including the femur, tibia, fibula, patella, tarsals, metatarsals, and phalanges
   The *pelvic girdle,* which is made up of the pelvic or coxal bones, sacrum, and coccyx.

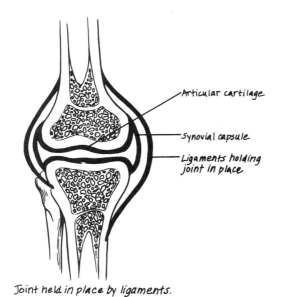

Articular cartilage

Synovial capsule

Ligaments holding joint in place

Joint held in place by ligaments.

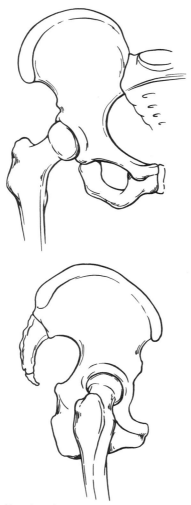

Ball and socket joint (hip joint-femur and coxal bones).

Axial Skeleton

- The *axial skeleton* includes the bones of the trunk, skull, vertebral column, ribs, sternum, and hyoid.

- The *skull* has 22 bones, and the *vertebral column* has 33 separate bones, however, the bones in the sacrum and coccyx are fused together. There are 12 pairs of ri*bs,* 1 *sternum,* and 1 *hyoid* bone, which is located in the neck.

JOINTS OF THE SKELETON

- Bones articulate to form joints which are held together by cartilage and ligaments. Joints are classified according to their movement.

- Joints are classified as synarthrosis, amphiarthrosis, and diarthrosis. *Synarthrosis* describes immovable joints such as the sutures in the skull. *Amphiarthrosis* refers to slightly movable joints with bone surfaces connected by fibrous cartilage disks or fibrous bands. This type of arrangement is found in the vertebral column, symphysis pubis, and tibiofibular joint. *Diarthrosis* or freely movable joints are articulations lined with synovial membranes and held in place by ligaments. Examples of diarthrosis are the knee, shoulder, hand, wrist, and ankle.

- The following types of movement are associated with diarthrodial joints

  A *ball-and-socket joint* has movement in all directions; examples are the shoulder and hip.

  A *hinge joint* is involved in flexion and extension where a concave surface articulates with a convex surface; examples of a hinge joint include the elbow and the phalanges in the hands and feet.

  A *gliding joint* has a sliding movement as one bone moves against another; examples are the wrist and ankle joints.

  A *pivot* joint has rotational movement; an example is the articulation between the radius and the ulna. As the hand is pronated, the head of the radius rotates and the shaft of the radius crosses over the ulna.

A *saddle joint* has movement in a variety of directions; an example is the articulation between the first finger (thumb) metacarpals and carpals.

A *condyloid joint* also has a variety of movements; examples are the joints between the metacarpals and phalanges.

BONES OF THE UPPER EXTREMITIES

- The bones of the upper extremities are the humerus, radius, ulna, wrist, hand (palm), and fingers (digits).

- The proximal *humerus* articulates with the scapula at the shoulder girdle and then distally with the radius and ulna at the elbow.

- The proximal portion of the humerus has expanded protuberances or prominences called greater and lesser tuberosities (tubercles). With the hand in the anatomical position the *greater tuberosity* is superior and lateral, forming the rounded prominence of the edge of the shoulder.

- The rounded *head* located on the proximal end of the humerus articulates with the glenoid fossa of the scapula, forming the shoulder joint. Just below the head is the *anatomical neck*.

- Inferior and medial to the greater tuberosity is the lesser tuberosity.

- The greater and lesser tuberosities serve as attachments for the muscles of the upper arm.

- Located between the greater and lesser tuberosities is the *bicipital* or *intertuberosity* (intertubercle) *groove*.

- Just inferior to the tuberosities is the *surgical neck,* so called because it is a frequent site of fractures of the upper humerus. The long diaphysis is the *shaft*.

- The distal end of the humerus has *medial* and *lateral condyles*. Above the condyles are rounded articular prominences called *medial* and *lateral epicondyles*. The epicondyle can be described as a small bump on the outer surface of the condyle.

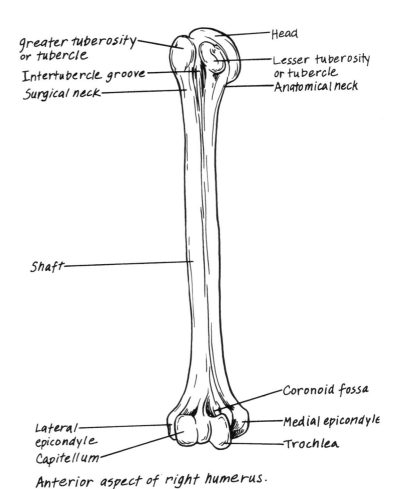

Anterior aspect of right humerus.

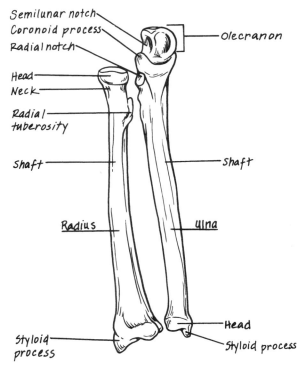

Anterior aspect of right radius and ulna.

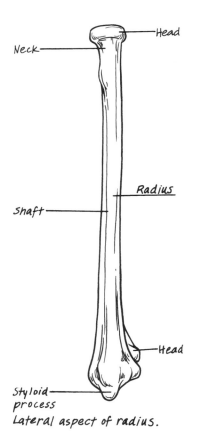

Lateral aspect of radius.

- The medial condyle has a smooth articular surface called the *trochlea*, and the lateral condyle has a smooth inner surface called the *capitellum*.

- On the anterior surface of the distal humerus is a small depression called the *coronoid fossa*.

- On the posterior surface of the distal humerus is a depression called the *olecranon fossa*.

Forearm

- The bones of the forearm are two long bones called the *radius* and *ulna*. The radius and ulna lie parallel to one another when the arm is in the anatomical position. As the hand is rotated medially, the distal end of the radius crosses over the ulna.

Radius

- The radius has an expanded proximal end with an almost flat surface on top. The expanded portion is the *head*, and the neck is just inferior to the head.

- On the medial surface just below the neck is the *radial tuberosity*.

- The long portion of the radius is called the *shaft*.

- On the lateral side of the distal radius is the pointed *styloid process*.

Ulna

- On the expanded proximal end of the ulna is a halfmoon-shaped notch called the *semilunar notch*. The most prominent posterior point or tip is known as the *olecranon process*.

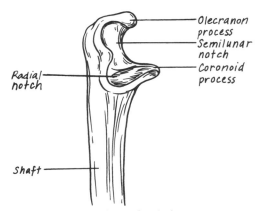

Lateral aspect of proximal ulna.

- On the lateral side of the semilunar notch is a depressed area called the *radial notch* which is involved in the articulation of the lateral aspect of the head of the radius.

- On the anterior aspect of the semilunar notch is a beaklike process called the *coronoid process.*

- The long portion of the ulna is called the *shaft.*

- The distal end of the ulna is slightly expanded, with a small projection called the *styloid process.*

Articulation of the Humerus and Forearm

- The head of the radius articulates with the capitellum, and the semilunar notch articulates with the trochlea.

- With the arm in the extended position, the olecranon process fits into the olecranon fossa.

- With the arm in the flexed position, the coronoid process fits into the coronoid fossa.

Bones of the Wrist

- There are eight small, irregularly shaped bones in the wrist aligned in two rows. These bones are

  Proximal row (from thumb side): navicular or scaphoid, lunate or semilunar, triquetrum or triangular, and pisiform
  Distal row (from thumb side): greater multangular or trapezium, lesser multangular or trapezoid, capitate or capitatum, and hamate or unciform.

Bones of the Hand

- The hand is composed of the bones of the palm or metacarpals and the digits or phalanges.

- There are five *metacarpals*, which are cylindrical in shape. Beginning on the lateral or thumb side they are recognized as the first through the fifth metacarpals.

- The *phalanges* are the bones of the fingers, with a total of 14 phalanges in the five digits (fingers).

- The first digit or thumb has only two phalanges, the *proximal phalanx*, and the *distal phalanx.*

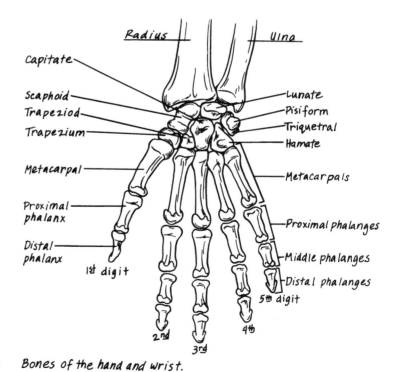

Bones of the hand and wrist.

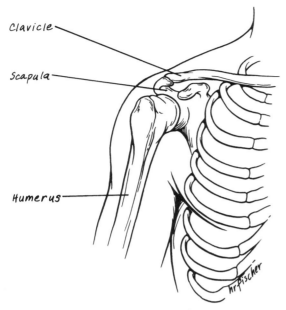

Anterior aspect of shoulder girdle.

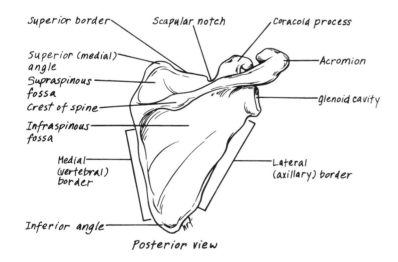

Posterior view

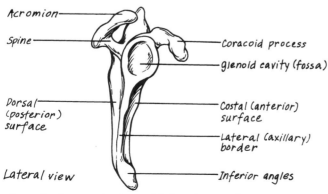

Lateral view

Scapula from posterior and lateral aspect.

- The second, third, fourth, and fifth digits are basically the same, having *proximal, middle,* and *distal phalanges*

The Shoulder Girdle

- The shoulder girdle provides support for the upper arm to connect to the trunk of the body. It is formed by two bones, the *scapula* (shoulder blade) and the *clavicle* (collarbone).

Scapula

- The glenoid fossa of the scapula articulates directly with the head of the humerus to form the shoulder joint.

- The scapula is a triangular, flat bone with a ridge arising from the upper medial posterior surface. The ridge becomes more prominent toward the lateral surface, with an expanded portion extending superiorly and laterally to the body of the scapula.

- The ridge is the *spine* of the scapula, and the more lateral expanded portion is the *acromion process.* The acromion process articulates with the clavicle.

- Superior to the scapular spine is the *supraspinous fossa.*

- Inferior to the scapular spine is the *infraspinous fossa.*

- The most lateral rounded portion is the *glenoid fossa* which is slightly concave. The glenoid fossa articulates directly with the humerus.

- Superior and anterior is an angled projection arising from the body of the scapula called the *coracoid process.*

- Across the superior border of the scapula is the *scapular notch.*

- The *superior medial angle* forms the curve on the upper medial surface.

- The most inferior portion of the scapula is the *inferior angle.*

- The anterior surface of the scapula is the costal surface and is slightly concave.

Clavicle

- The *clavicle* is a long bone with a slight curve.

- The medial end of the clavicle is slightly expanded to become the *sternal* extremity and is the part that articulates with the sternum.

- The lateral aspect is slightly larger and is called the *acromion extremity*; it articulates with the acromion process of the scapula.

THE BONES OF THE LOWER EXTREMITIES

- The bones of the lower extremities are the femur, patella, tibia, fibula, tarsals, metatarsals, and phalanges.

Femur (Thigh)

- The longest and strongest bone in the body is the *femur*.

- The shape of the femur is very similar to that of the humerus, but it has a longer, thicker shaft and larger prominences on both the proximal and distal ends.

- At the most proximal point on the femur is the rounded *head*.

- The head of the femur articulates with the pelvic bone to form the hip joint.

- Just inferior to the head is the more narrow *neck*.

- Inferior and lateral to the neck is a large eminence or projection called the *greater trochanter*.

- More posterior and medial is the *lesser trochanter*. A ridge called the *intertrochanteric crest* runs from the greater and lesser trochanters on the proximal posterior surface.

- The long portion of the femur is the *shaft*.

- Two eminences or protuberances are present at the distal end. They are the *medial* and *lateral condyles*.

- Lying just above the condyles are the *medial* and *lateral epicondyles*.

- Between the two condyles on the distal posterior surface of the femur is a significant depression called the *intercondyloid fossa*.

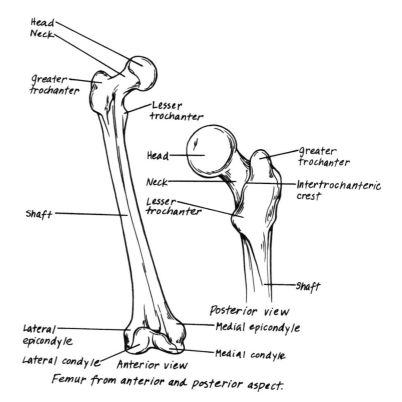

Femur from anterior and posterior aspect.

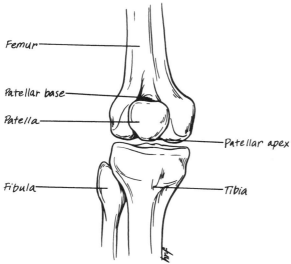

Knee joint demonstrating position of patella.

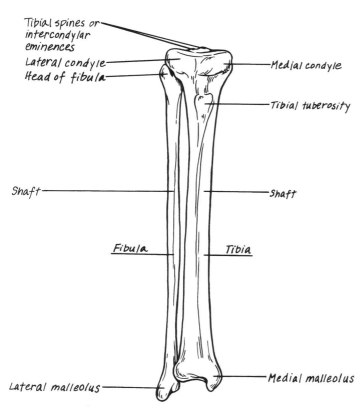

Anterior aspect of tibia and fibula.

Patella

- The *patella* is the largest sesamoid bone in the body.

- The patella lies at a level just superior to the knee joint.

- The patella develops in the tendons of the leg where it is held in place by ligaments.

- The most superior border of the patella is the *base*, and the most inferior border is the *apex*.

The Lower Leg

- The bones of the lower leg are the *tibia* and *fibula*, which are parallel to one another.

Tibia

- The *tibia* is the larger bone and is positioned more medially.

- The tibia has a long *shaft* and two expanded portions on the proximal and distal ends.

- The expanded end of the tibia has two projections called the *medial* and *lateral condyles*.

- The surface across the top of the tibia is quite flat and is called the *tibial plateau*. It has two small, pointed tips projecting upward which are known as *tibial spines* or *intercondyloid eminences*.

- On the distal and medial portions of the tibia is the *medial malleolus*.

- The lateral surface of the distal tibia is flatter, forming an articulation with the fibula.

Fibula

- The *fibula* is the lateral long bone in the lower leg. It is a slender bone with slightly expanded ends.

- The long portion of the fibula is the *shaft*.

- The most proximal point on the fibula is the *styloid process*. Just inferior to the styloid process is the *head*.

- The expanded distal end of the fibula is the *lateral malleolus*.

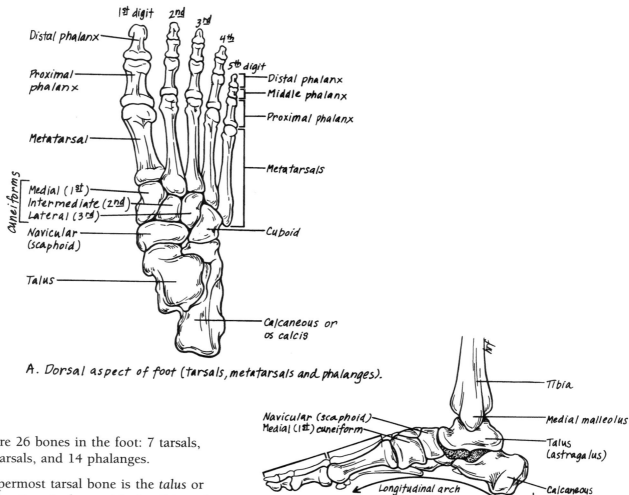

A. Dorsal aspect of foot (tarsals, metatarsals and phalanges).

B. Medial aspect of lateral foot and ankle.

The Foot

- There are 26 bones in the foot: 7 tarsals, 5 metatarsals, and 14 phalanges.

- The uppermost tarsal bone is the *talus* or *astragalus*. It articulates with the tibia and fibula to form the ankle joint.

- Inferior and posterior to the talus is the largest of the tarsal bones, the *os calcis* or *calcaneus*, which forms the heel of the foot.

- Anterior to the talus is the *navicular* or *scaphoid*.

- Anterior to the navicular are four bones called the cuneiforms and the cuboid. These four bones form the *transverse arch* of the foot. Beginning on the medial side is the *medial* or *first cuneiform*, the *middle* or *second cuneiform*, and the *lateral* or *third cuneiform*. Lateral to the cuneiforms is the *cuboid*.

- Articulating distally to the cuneiforms and cuboid are the five *metatarsals*. The first metatarsal is on the medial side, with the fifth metatarsal most lateral.

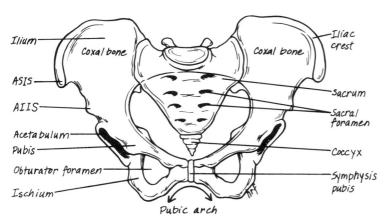

Anterior aspect of pelvis (coxal bones, sacrum and coccyx).

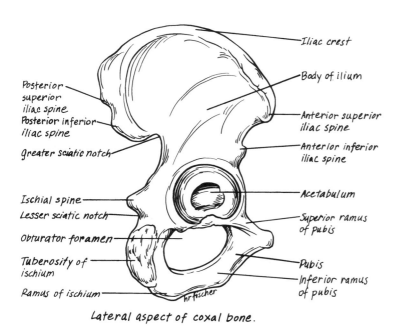

Lateral aspect of coxal bone.

- The metatarsals and tarsals form the *longitudinal arches* of the foot, which extend from the calcaneus to the head of the metatarsals.

- The phalanges are distributed in the same way as in the fingers. The first digit (big toe) has only two phalanges, called the *proximal* and *distal phalanges.*

- The second through fifth digits each have *proximal, middle,* and *distal phalanges.*

The Pelvic Girdle

- The bones of the pelvis form a basin with an oval or round opening. The pelvic girdle supports the trunk and connects the lower extremities to the body.

- The bones that form the pelvic basin are the two *coxal* bones (forming the hipbone), the *sacrum,* and the *coccyx.* (The sacrum and coccyx will be reviewed along with the veterbral column in Chapter 4.)

Coxal Bone

- The coxal bone is actually three bones fused together.

- The upper, fan-shaped bone is the *ilium.* At the most superior point of the ilium is the *iliac crest.* Anterior is a pointed prominence called the *anterior superior iliac spine* (ASIS), and just inferior to the ASIS is a lesser prominence called the *anterior inferior iliac spine* (AIIS).

- Prominences on the posterior edge of the ilium are referred to as the *posterior superior iliac spine* (PSIS) and the *posterior inferior iliac spine* (PIIS).

- The fused bone lying inferior and anterior to the ilium is the *pubis.* Extending superiorly and slightly laterally is the *superior ramus* of the pubis. Inferior and slightly lateral is the *inferior ramus* of the pubis which forms part of the inferior border of the obturator foramen. The superior ramus of the pubis forms part of the upper border of the obturator foramen.

- The posterior and inferior portions of the coxal bone are called the *ischium*. Extending from the body of the ischium are the ischial rami, which join the pubis bone to the borders of the obturator foramen.

- The large bump on the posterior inferior surface of the ischium is known as the *ischial tuberosity*, the weight-bearing point when a person is sitting. Superior to the ischial tuberosity is the *ischial spine*.

- The ilium, pubis, and ischium are fused together to form a large cavity called the *acetabulum*.

- The acetabulum is a large concave area that holds the head of the femur to form the hip joint.

- The two pubic bones join in the midsagittal line anteriorly to form the *symphysis pubis*.

- The rami of the symphysis pubis and ischium form a circle around an opening called the *obturator foramen*.

- The two coxal bones articulate posteriorly with the sacrum to form an oval basin.

- The upper border of the pelvic basin is the pelvic inlet, and the lower border is the pelvic outlet. In the female pelvis the open passageway between the pelvic inlet and the pelvic outlet form part of the birth canal.

Characteristics of the Pelvis in the Male and Female

- The shape of the pelvis differs in the male and female, resulting in distinct characteristics in each case.

- The *male pelvis* is characteristically more vertical. Bones appear to be thicker, the obturator foramen is larger, the acetabulum is larger, the pelvic cavity is more narrow, the sacrum is more narrow, and there is less movement of the coccyx.

- The *female pelvis* is characteristically broad and shallow. Bones appear lighter, the obturator foramen is small, the acetabulum is small, the sacrum is wider, the coccyx is more flexible, and the angle of the pubic arch is greater.

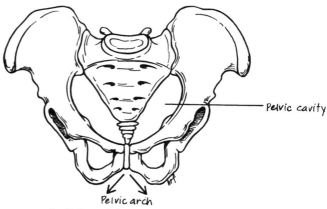

Pelvic cavity

Pelvic arch

A. Male pelvis.
Comparison in shape between male and female pelvis.

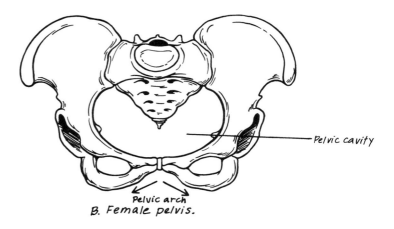

Pelvic cavity

Pelvic arch
B. Female pelvis.

PATHOPHYSIOLOGIC TERMINOLOGY ASSOCIATED WITH BONE TISSUE AND THE APPENDICULAR SKELETON

Acromegaly enlargement of the bones of the extremities and the soft tissue of the face; this condition may result from abnormal secretion of growth hormone by the pituitary gland

Chondritis an inflammation of cartilaginous tissue

Exostosis abnormal bone growth

Fracture a crack or a complete break in a bone of the skeleton

Colles' fracture a (usually complete) fracture to the distal end of the radius with bone displacement

Comminuted fracture a complete fracture, with the bone splintered at the site of impact

Complete fracture a complete break through the entire bone

Compound fracture a complete fracture, with the bone breaking through the soft tissue and skin

Displaced fracture a complete fracture, with the bones at the site of the fracture out of alignment

Greenstick fracture a type of fracture seen in children where the fracture is not complete and the bone begins to bend slightly.

Impacted fracture a complete fracture, with the broken ends jammed into each other

Incomplete fracture a fracture that does not go through the entire bone

Pathologic fracture a fracture of a bone that has been weakened by osteoporosis or cancer; may occur spontaneously or without trauma to the area

Spiral fracture a fracture in which the fracture line has a spiral appearance; usually results from severe twisting of the bone

Stress fracture a fracture that may occur in the metatarsals of the foot as a result of repeated stress during rigorous training or running long distances

Gout an excessive amount of uric acid in the blood producing crystallized deposits in joints, kidneys, and soft tissue

Osteitis inflammation of bone tissue

Osteoarthritis a degenerative joint disease producing pain and stiffness, usually due to aging, wear, and tear

Osteogenesis imperfecta a condition in which bones are brittle and fracture easily

Osteoma a tumor of bone tissue

Osteosarcoma a malignant tumor of bone tissue

Rheumatoid arthritis an inflammatory process
affecting the joints and producing swelling,
pain, and degeneration of the joint; the origin
may be autoimmune
Sprain twisting of a joint with some displacement of the support structure holding the
joint in place
Synovitis inflammation of a joint.

Chapter 3 Practice Questions

1. The end of a long bone is called
   a. the epiphysis.
   b. the diaphysis.
   c. the medulla.
   d. cancellous bone.

2. Cells that form bone tissue are
   a. osteocytes.
   b. osteoclasts.
   c. osteoblasts.
   d. the periosteum.

3. The membrane covering bones except for their articular surfaces is called
   a. the articular cartilage.
   b. an osteoblast.
   c. an osteoclast.
   d. the periosteum.

4. Which of the following is the type of bone tissue that produces red blood cells?
   a. hard, compact bone
   b. cancellous bone
   c. epiphyseal disk
   d. medulla bone marrow

5. A ball-and-socket movement demonstrates which type of joint?
   a. synarthrosis
   b. amphiarthrosis
   c. diarthrosis
   d. fibrocartilage

6. Which of the following is an example of a synarthrodial joint?
   a. the symphysis pubis
   b. the vertebral column
   c. the sutures of the skull
   d. the ankle joint

7. The proximal humerus articulates with the _____ of the _____.
   a. acromion process, clavicle
   b. glenoid fossa, scapula
   c. head, radius
   d. olecranon process, ulna

8. The greater and lesser tuberosities are located on the _____ of the _____.
   a. proximal end, humerus
   b. distal end, humerus
   c. proximal end, femur
   d. distal end, femur

9. Located between the greater and lesser tuberosities is the
   a. surgical neck.
   b. anatomical neck.
   c. diaphysis.
   d. bicipital or intertubercle groove.

10. The coronoid fossa is part of which bone?
    a. ulna
    b. radius
    c. scapula
    d. humerus

11. At the proximal end the head of the radius articulates with the
    a. capitellum.
    b. trochlea.
    c. olecranon fossa.
    d. coronoid fossa.

12. Which of the following lists of bones represents the correct alignment of the carpal bones beginning on the thumb side, proximal row?
    a. greater multangular, unciform, pisiform, capitatum
    b. navicular, lunate, pisiform, unciform
    c. pisiform, triquetrum, lunate, navicular
    d. navicular, lunate, triquetrum, pisiform

13. The palm of the hand is formed by which set of bones?
    a. carpals
    b. metacarpals
    c. sesamoids
    d. phalanges

14. The fingers or digits are formed by which set of bones?
    a. carpals   c. sesamoids
    b. metacarpals   d. phalanges

15. The shoulder girdle is formed by which of the following bones?
    a. clavicle, scapula, and ribs
    b. clavicle, scapula, and humerus
    c. clavicle, scapula, and upper extremity
    d. clavicle and scapula

16. The lateral expanded projection of the scapula that articulates with the clavicle is the
    a. spine of the scapula.
    b. acromion process.
    c. coracoid process.
    d. scapular notch.

17. The longest and strongest bone in the body is the
    a. femur.
    b. vertebral column.
    c. humerus.
    d. tibia.

18. The most proximal portion of the femur that articulates with the pelvic girdle is the
    a. acetabulum.
    b. greater trochanter.
    c. lesser trochanter.
    d. head.

19. The two large eminences on the distal end of the femur are the
    a. medial and lateral condyles.
    b. medial and lateral trochanters.
    c. intercondyloid eminences.
    d. intercondyloid fossae.

20. Which of the following is the largest and most posterior bone in the foot?
    a. talus   c. cuneiform
    b. os calcis   d. cuboid

21. The three bones fused together to form the coxal bone are the
    a. ileum, pubis, and ischium.
    b. ilium, pubis, and ischium.
    c. ischium, acetabulum, and pubis.
    d. ischium, ilium, and acetabulum.

22. The anterior and superior prominence on the ilium is the
    a. iliac ramus.
    b. ala or wing.
    c. ASIS.
    d. AIIS.

23. The bone(s) forming the acetabulum is (are) the
    a. ilium.
    b. ilium and pubis.
    c. ischium.
    d. ilium, ischium, and pubis.

24. **The type of fracture involving a complete break in the bone and splintering of the bone at the site of impact is called**

    a. a complete fracture.
    b. a compound fracture.
    c. a comminuted fracture.
    d. an impacted fracture.

25. **An inflammatory process of the joints accompanied by swelling and pain is called**

    a. arthritis.
    b. rheumatoid arthritis.
    c. osteoarthritis.
    d. synovitis.

The Skeleton: Part Two
Bones of the
Axial Skeleton

- The bones of the *axial skeleton* are the *thoracic cage*, *vertebral column*, and *skull*.

THE THORACIC CAGE

- The bones of the *thoracic cage* are 12 pairs of *ribs*, 12 thoracic *vertebrae*, and the *sternum*.

- The upper 10 pairs of ribs have *costal cartilage* on the anterior aspect for attachment to the sternum.

- The shape of the ribs combined with the presence of costal cartilage allows for movement facilitating expansion of the lungs during breathing. (The vertebrae will be reviewed along with the vertebral column later in this chapter.)

Ribs

- There are 12 pairs of *ribs* attached posteriorly to the thoracic vertebrae and anteriorly to costal cartilage that articulates with the sternum.

- The upper 7 pairs of ribs are called *true ribs*. Each pair articulates posteriorly with a thoracic vertebra and anteriorly with costal cartilage directly attached to the sternum.

- The lower 5 pairs of ribs are called *false ribs*. They articulate posteriorly with a thoracic vertebra and anteriorly with costal cartilage but do not directly articulate with the sternum.

- The lower 2 pairs of ribs are called *floating* ribs. They are short and thin and have no attachment to cartilage or to the sternum.

- Ribs are long, thin, flat bones with an expanded portion on the posterior aspect called the *head*.

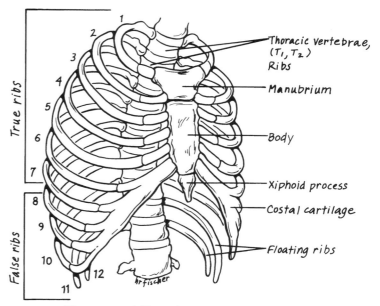

Rib cage and thoracic vertebrae.

- Next to the head is the *neck* and a bump called the rib *tuberosity.*

- The head articulates with the body of a thoracic vertebra, and the tuberosity articulates with the transverse process of the thoracic vertebra.

- Ribs are C-shaped with all articulations intact, forming a protective cage around the lungs and pleural cavity.

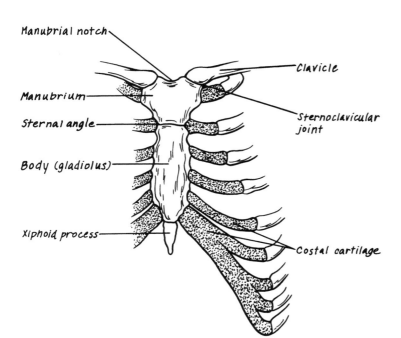

Manubrial notch

Clavicle

Manubrium

Sternoclavicular joint

Sternal angle

Body (gladiolus)

Xiphoid process

Costal cartilage

Sternum with costal cartilage and clavicle articulation.

Sternum

- The *sternum,* also called the *breastbone,* lies anteriorly to and receives the articulations of the ribs and clavicle.

- The sternum is a narrow, flat bone and has three sections.

- The uppermost, broadest section of the sternum is the *manubrium.* The costal cartilage of the first pair of ribs articulates directly with the lateral aspect of the manubrium.

- In the most superior region of the manubrium is a notch called the *manubrial notch.* This notch is easily palpated and is used as an anatomic landmark for positioning of the body.

- The middle and longest part of the sternum is the *body* or *gladiolus.*

- The *sternal angle* is a prominence where the body articulates with the sternum.

- Six pairs of rib cartilage articulate directly with the body of the sternum.

- The costal cartilage attached to the lower pairs of ribs does not articulate with the sternum but is attached to the cartilage of the nearest superior rib.

- The lowermost portion of the sternum is the *xiphoid process.* It is small and is composed mostly of cartilage.

- Like the manubrial notch, the xiphoid process is used as a positioning landmark.

- The *manubrial notch* usually lies at the level of the *intervertebral space* between T2 and T3 when the body is in the erect position.

- The xiphoid process is usually at the level of the tenth thoracic vertebra when the body is in the erect position.

- The sternum also articulates with the clavicles at the manubrial angles, which are on either side of the manubrial notch.

- The joints formed by articulation of the sternum and clavicle are known as the *sterno-clavicular joints.*

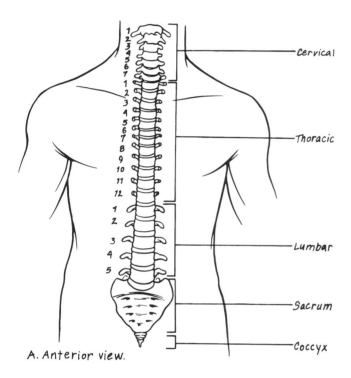

A. Anterior view.

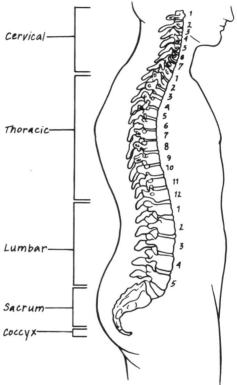

B. Lateral view.
Anterior (A) and lateral (B) aspects of vertebral column.

BONES OF THE VERTEBRAL COLUMN

- The *vertebral column* has 33 vertebrae, with the vertebrae of the sacrum and coccyx fused together.

- The vertebral column serves as the support structure for the body and encloses the spinal cord.

- The vertebral column lies in the midline or midsagittal plane and is on the posterior surface of the body.

- The bones that compose the vertebral column are 7 cervical vertebrae, 12 thoracic vertebrae, 5 lumbar vertebrae, 5 fused vertebrae forming the sacrum, and 4 fused vertebrae forming the coccyx.

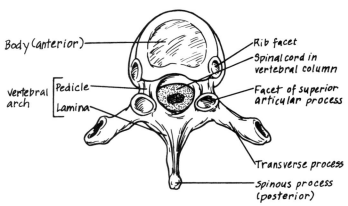

Superior aspect of typical vertebra.

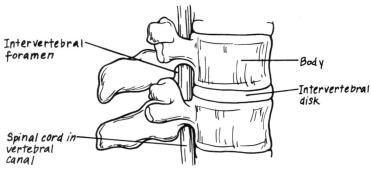

Vertebrae with intervertebral disk.

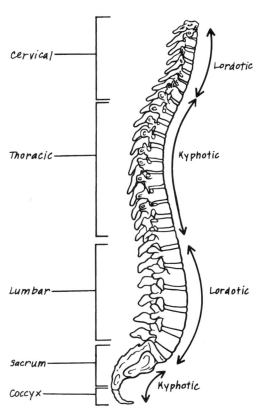

Normal curvatures for vertebral column.

- Each segment or section has unique characteristics. Vertebrae lying adjacent to another section take on similar characteristics such as the body becoming larger or smaller and the transverse and spinous processes becoming shorter or longer. A typical vertebra has a *body, pedicles, transverse processes, laminae, a spinous process,* and *articular facets.*

- The smallest vertebrae are the *cervical* vertebrae, which are at the top of the vertebral column.

- The *thoracic* vertebrae are slightly larger and increase in size near the next section which is the lumbar section.

- The *lumbar* vertebrae are larger and have a large vertebral body.

- The two lowermost sections are fused vertebrae known as the *sacrum* and *coccyx.*

- Other characteristics unique to each section are the location of the articular facets and intervertebral foramina. For example, the *transverse foramina* are found only in the cervical vertebrae.

- Located between the body of each vertebra is an *intervertebral disk.*

- The intervertebral disk has a thick, fibrous covering known as the *annulus fibrosus.* The annulus fibrosus encloses a soft, jellylike center called the *nucleus pulposus.*

- Intervertebral disks serve as cushions for the vertebrae as they articulate with one another, facilitating movement of the vertebral column.

- The vertebral column has natural curves which develop in childhood.

- The curve of the cervical and lumbar sections is convex and is called a *lordotic curve.*

- The curve of the thoracic, sacrum, and coccyx is concave and is called a *kyphotic curve.*

- These curves facilitate balance, posture, and movement.

- Although the specific anatomy may vary, an arch is formed just posterior to the body of the vertebra.

- The arch encircles what is called the *vertebral foramen* and is formed by the body anteriorly; the pedicles and lamina form the posterior portion of the arch.

- The *spinal cord* and *nerves* branching from the spinal cord are located within the vertebral foramen which forms a canal structure within the vertebral column. The vertebral canal encloses the spinal cord and the associated branching nerves.

- As two vertebrae articulate with an intervertebral disk in between them, an *intervertebral foramen* is formed. On its lateral side nerves pass from the spinal cord through the intervertebral foramen to peripheral parts of the body.

Cervical Vertebrae

- There are seven *cervical vertebrae* called C1 through C7.

- The cervical vertebrae articulate with the base of the cranium and with the thoracic vertebrae to form the neck.

- One unique characteristic of the cervical vertebrae is the *transverse foramen* which is an opening in each of the *transverse processes* for a major blood vessel to pass through.

- In addition, vertebrae C1 and C2 have other unique characteristics.

- *C1* is not a typical vertebra. It is called the *atlas* because it is the most superior vertebra and "holds up" the cranium as it articulates with the occipital bone.

- C1 has no body and has larger expanded articular facets as part of the lateral masses. There is an anterior arch and a posterior arch enclosing a larger vertebral foramen.

- The transverse processes are short, and each has a transverse foramen.

- C2, the *axis*, is the second cervical vertebra and has its own unique characteristics.

- The body of C2 is small and has a toothlike projection which rises superiorly to articulate with the posterior wall of the anterior arch on C1.

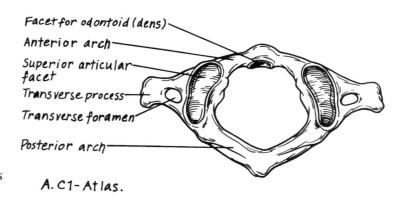

Facet for odontoid (dens)
Anterior arch
Superior articular facet
Transverse process
Transverse foramen
Posterior arch

A. C1- Atlas.

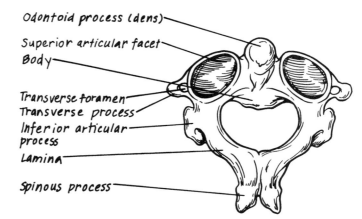

Odontoid process (dens)
Superior articular facet
Body
Transverse foramen
Transverse process
Inferior articular process
Lamina
Spinous process

B. C2-Axis.
A) First cervical (atlas) vertebra and B) second cervical (axis) vertebra.

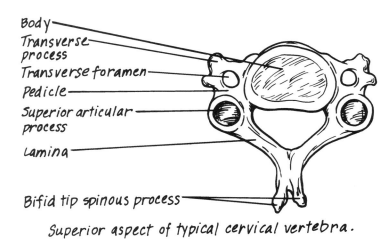

Superior aspect of typical cervical vertebra.

Rib attachments to thoracic vertebrae.

- The projection rising from C2 is the *odontoid process* or *dens,* which facilitates turning of the head from one side to the other.

- The transverse processes are thick and have *superior* and *inferior articular processes.*

- *C3* through *C6* are typical cervical vertebrae; they are small and have short, spinous processes with *bifid* (two-pronged) *tips.*

- *C7* has an extremely long, prominent spinous process called the *vertebra prominens* and can be easily palpated externally at the base of the neck.

- The transverse processes extend laterally from the vertebral body and have *transverse foramina* on both sides.

- The *pedicle* is very short. An enlarged area is present as the pedicle and *laminae* come together, giving rise to the superior and inferior articular processes.

- Where the cervical vertebrae join together, the intervertebral foramen lies at an angle of 45 degrees to the anterior aspect of the midsagittal plane. This corresponds to the amount the body must be rotated when being positioned to demonstrate the intervertebral foramina of the cervical section of the vertebral column.

- The articulations between the vertebrae form joints called *apophyseal joints.*

- The apophyseal joints lie at right angles to the midsagittal plane. To demonstrate the apophyseal joints of the cervical vertebrae, the body must be rotated 90 degrees from the midsagittal plane.

Thoracic Vertebrae

- There are 12 *thoracic vertebrae* known as T1 through T2.

- The thoracic vertebrae are larger in size than the cervical vertebrae.

- The transverse processes are longer and are directed inferiorly. In general, thoracic vertebrae have longer spinal processes than cervical vertebrae.

- T11 and T12 begin to increase in size and take on more of the appearance of lumbar vertebrae.

- Thoracic vertebrae are more typical in shape, with a large body and *pedicles* extending posteriorly, giving rise to the transverse processes.

- The *laminae* join posteriorly to give rise to the spinous process.

- The transverse processes of the thoracic vertebrae have a slight posterior tilt, with the unique characteristic of facets for ribs on the anterior surface.

- The *intervertebral foramina* of the thoracic vertebrae lie at a 90-degree angle from the midsagittal plane and can be radiographically demonstrated with the same amount of rotation of the body.

- The *apophyseal joints* of the thoracic vertebrae lie at an angle 70 degrees from the midsagittal plane.

- To demonstrate the apophyseal joints, the body must be rotated 70 degrees from the midsagittal plane, or it can be rotated 20 degrees anteriorly from the lateral position of the vertebrae.

Lumbar Vertebrae

- There are five *lumbar* vertebrae known as L1 through L5.

- The lumbar vertebrae have a round, thick body which is the largest body of all the vertebrae.

- The *pedicle* arises from the posterior and lateral aspects of the body of the vertebra.

- The *transverse processes* extend laterally from the posterior border of the pedicles.

- The transverse process is shorter than in the thoracic vertebrae.

- The *lamina*, which forms the posterior border of the vertebral foramen, extends from the transverse processes to form the *spinous process*.

- The spinous processes of the lumbar section are large and almost rectangular compared to those of the other vertebral groups.

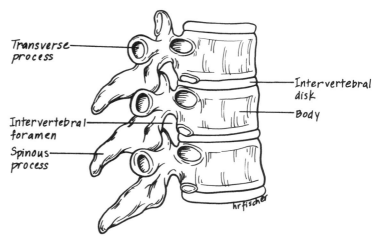

Thoracic intervertebral foramina demonstrated by joining thoracic vertebrae.

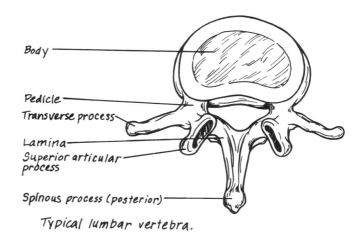

Typical lumbar vertebra.

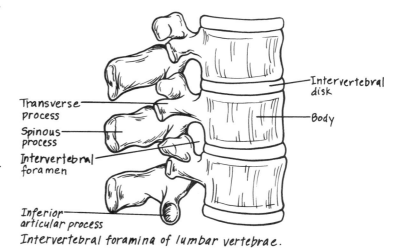

Intervertebral foramina of lumbar vertebrae.

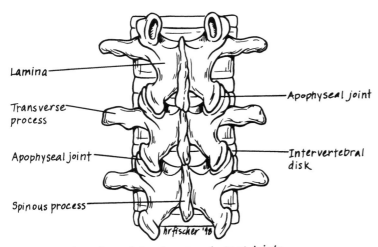

Posterior view of lumbar apophyseal joints.

- Extending from the junction of the transverse process and lamina are the *superior articular* and *inferior articular processes.*

- The lower lumbar vertebrae, especially L5, have a broader body and appear more wedge-shaped as they articulate with the sacrum.

- The lumbar *intervertebral foramen* is a round opening formed by the joining of two vertebrae. The intervertebral foramina in the lumbar vertebrae lie at an angle of 90 degrees to the midsagittal plane; therefore the same amount of body rotation is required to demonstrate these articulations on radiographic images.

- The lumbar *apophyseal joints* lie at an angle of 30 to 45 degrees posteriorly to the midsagittal plane.

- To demonstrate the apophyseal joints of the upper and midlumbar regions body rotation should be approximately 45 degrees.

- To demonstrate the apophyseal joints of the lower and lumbosacral junction the body rotation should be about 35 degrees.

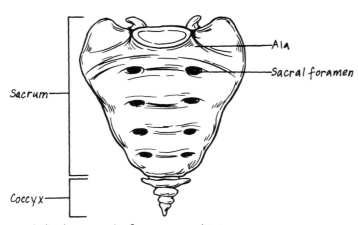

Anterior aspect of sacrum and coccyx.

Sacrum

- The *sacrum* is formed by five fused vertebrae and serves as a major support for the entire vertebral column.

- The sacrum is triangular in shape with bilateral openings called *sacral foramina.*

- Sacral foramina allow blood vessels and nerves to extend through to the lower parts of the body.

- The anterior and superior border of the body of the sacrum is a sharp lip known as the *sacral promontory.*

- The fused transverse processes of the sacrum form the *sacral ala.*

- The natural curve of the sacrum is concave forward.

Coccyx

- The *coccyx* is composed of four small fused vertebrae. In females the coccyx is more flexible, especially during childbirth.

- The width and size of the coccygeal segments become smaller from the first to the fourth segment.

BONES OF THE SKULL

- The bones of the skull are divided into two categories: cranial bones and facial bones.

- There are 8 *cranial bones* that enclose the brain and 14 facial bones that form the face, orbits, nasal cavity, and chin.

- The bones of the skull are joined together by *sutures,* which are synarthrodial or immovable joints.

- At birth the cranial bones are not fully developed. At the points where the cranial bones are joined together there are fibrous membranes called *fontanelles.* The fontanelles allow for some movement between the bones as the infant skull passes through the birth canal. The fontanelles close as the skull develops, forming sutures.

- The *anterior fontanelle* is near the vertex or bregma of the skull and is formed by the joining of the frontal and two parietal bones. The sphenoid and mastoid fontanelles are on the lateral aspects of the skull.

- The *sphenoid fontanelle* is formed by the joining of the frontal, sphenoid, and parietal bones.

- The *mastoid fontanelle* is formed by the joining of the temporal, parietal, and occipital bones.

- The *posterior fontanelle* is formed by the joining of the two parietal and occipital bones.

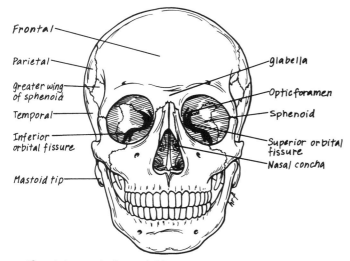

Frontal aspect of cranial bones.

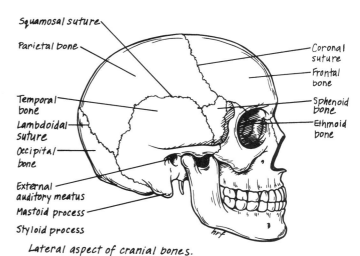

Lateral aspect of cranial bones.

The Cranium

- There are eight *cranial* bones called the frontal, parietal (right and left), sphenoid, temporal (right and left), occipital, and ethmoid.

Frontal Bone

- The *frontal bone* forms the forehead, anterior cranial cavity, and roof of the orbits.

- A curved arch, called the *superciliary arch,* is located just above the *supraorbital margin.*

- Between the superciliary arches is a slight prominence called the *glabella.*

- Immediately above each of the supraorbital margins is a *supraorbital foramen,* an opening that allows the passage of blood vessels and nerves.

- Embedded within the area behind the glabella and above the supraorbital area are paired *frontal sinuses.* These sinuses are air-filled cavities which provide resonance in speech.

- On the inferior surface of the frontal bones is a U-shaped opening called the *ethmoid notch.*

- The curved body of the frontal bone that forms the forehead is called the *squamous portion.*

Ethmoid Bone

- The *ethmoid bone* lies inferior to the frontal bone and anterior to the sphenoid bone; it articulates with the frontal bone at the ethmoid notch.

- The upper flat or horizontal portion is the *cribriform plate* and has pointed projections extending upward called *cristae galli.*

- At the midline of the ethmoid bone is the *vertical portion* or *perpendicular plate.*

- On either side of the perpendicular plate is a bony, air-filled section known as the *labyrinth.* The labyrinth forms part of the wall of the nasal cavity.

- Extending downward from the medial walls of the labyrinth are the *nasal chonchae.*

Parietal Bones

- Posterior to the frontal bone are the two *parietal bones* forming the superior and lateral walls of the cranium and the upper part of the cranial cavity.

- The parietal bones are rectangular, with a concave inner surface that forms the top of the skull.

- The suture formed by articulation of the frontal and anterior portions of the parietal bones is the *coronal suture.*

- The two parietal bones join together on the top of the skull to form the *sagittal suture* in the midsagittal plane.

Sphenoid Bone

- The *sphenoid bone* is quite irregular in shape and articulates with most of the cranial bones.

- The floor of the middle and anterior cranial cavity is formed by most of the main *body* of the sphenoid bone.

- Located on the central and superior surfaces of the sphenoid bone is the *sella turcica.* From the lateral aspect, the sella turcica looks like a saddle; it contains the pituitary gland which is part of the endocrine system.

- The anterior portion of the saddle has prominent points on each side called *anterior clinoid processes.*

- Posteriorly, the saddle has prominences called *posterior clinoid processes.*

- The posterior sloped surface of the posterior clinoid processes is the *dorsum sella.*

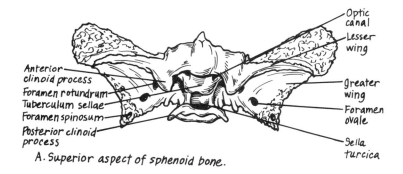

A. Superior aspect of sphenoid bone.

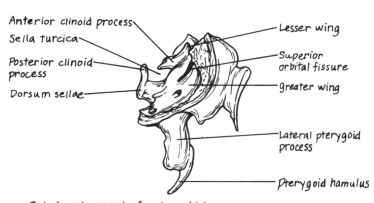

B. Lateral aspect of sphenoid bone.

- Extending laterally from the sella turcica are the *great wings* of the sphenoid.

- Arising from the anterior borders of the great wings are the *lesser wings* which extend posteriorly to form the anterior clinoid processes.

- At slightly oblique angles from the anterior aspect of the sella turcica are the right and left *optic foramen* and *superior orbital fissures.*

- Openings on the great wings are the *foramen rotundum, foramen ovale,* and *foramen spinosum.*

- Extending inferiorly and posteriorly from the great wings are the *pterygoid processes* and the *pterygoid hamulus.*

- On the lower part of the sphenoid bone are the *sphenoid sinuses,* which are paired cavities located beneath the sella turcica.

- Articulations of the sphenoid bone are the frontal and ethmoid bones on the anterior surface, the temporal and parietal bones on the lateral surfaces, and the occipital bone on the posterior surface. The sphenoid bone is the only bone that articulates with each of the cranial bones.

Temporal Bones

- The two *temporal bones* are located on the lateral inferior surfaces of the cranial cavity.

- The temporal bone is irregularly shaped, with a flat upper *squamous portion* forming the lower lateral wall of the cranium.

- Externally and on the lower surface is an opening called the *external auditory meatus,* which leads to the structures of the ear and hearing organs.

- Posterior and inferior to the external auditory meatus is a cone-shaped projection filled with air cells called the *mastoid process.*

- Slightly medial and inferior is a long, thin projection known as the *styloid process* of the temporal bone.

- The *zygomatic process* begins as a ridge rising from the external surface of the temporal bone just superior to the external auditory meatus.

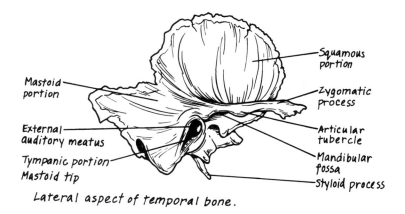

Lateral aspect of temporal bone.

- The zygomatic process joins with the projection from the zygoma (facial bone) to form the zygomatic arch.

- A dense bone extends medially and anteriorly at a 45-degree angle and is known as the *petrous portion* or *petrous ridge.*

- Located within the petrous ridge are the *middle* and *inner ear structures.* (The middle and inner ear structures will be reviewed as part of the sensory system.)

Occipital Bone

- The most posterior bone of the cranium is the *occipital bone.* It forms the posterior and base of the cranial cavity.

- From the lateral aspect the occipital bone forms a C-shape as part of the cranial cavity.

- Superiorly, the occipital bone articulates with the two parietal bones to form the *lambdoidal suture.*

- On the lower surface is a large opening called the *foramen magnum,* which contains the lower portion of the brainstem or medulla oblongata.

- Anterior to the foramen magnum is the *basilar portion* which articulates with the sphenoid bone. The interior surface of the basilar portion, forming a sloped surface as it articulates with the sphenoid, is the *clivus.*

- Extending inferiorly to either side of the foramen magnum are the *articular processes* or *condyles* which articulate with the first cervical vertebra.

- Posterior to the articular condyles and on either side of the foramen magnum are the *jugular foramina.*

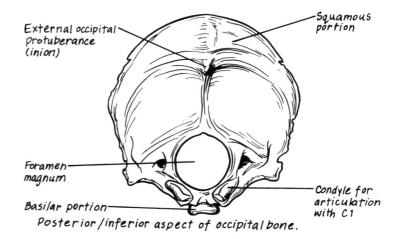

Posterior/inferior aspect of occipital bone.

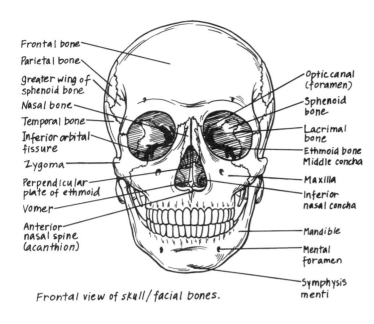

Frontal view of skull/facial bones.

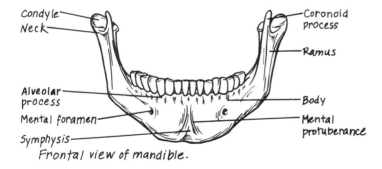

Frontal view of mandible.

The Facial Bones

- There are 14 bones that compose the face and jaw: the *mandible, lacrimal* (right and left), *maxilla* (right and left), *palatine* (right and left), *nasal* (right and left), *inferior nasal conchae* (right and left), *zygoma* (right and left), and *vomer*.

Mandible

- The largest and most dense facial bone is the *mandible*.

- The mandible forms part of the *temporo-mandibular joint* and is the only bone of the skull that moves.

- The mandible has a horseshoe shape, with a *ramus* extending superiorly at the posterior aspect. The ramus is flat, with a beaklike process on the anterior aspect called the *coronoid process* and a *condyle* for articulation on the posterior aspect.

- The central portion of the body is the mandibular *symphysis*.

- The inferior border at the symphysis is quite prominent and is known as the *mental protuberance*.

- On the superior surface of the U-shaped body of the mandible is the *alveolar process* where the roots of teeth are located.

Maxilla Bones

- The two *maxillae* are the largest of the remaining facial bones.

- The maxilla forms part of the wall and floor of the nasal cavity and the air-filled cavity, the *maxillary sinus*.

- The maxilla also forms most of the roof of the mouth.

Nasal Bones

- The *nasal bones* are two very small bones that articulate with each other to form the bridge of the nose.

- These bones articulate superiorly with the frontal bone and laterally with maxilla bones.

Zygoma Bones

- The two *zygoma bones* form the cheeks of the face.

- The zygoma articulates with the temporal bone to form the zygomatic arch.

- The lateral and inferior border of the orbit is formed by the zygoma.

Lacrimal Bones

- The two *lacrimal bones* form the anterior medial wall of the orbit and contain the lacrimal sacs or tear ducts.

- The lacrimal bones articulate with the labyrinth of the ethmoid bone and with the maxillae.

Palatine Bones

- The *palatine bones* are L-shaped bones that make up the posterior portion of the roof of the mouth and a small portion of the posterior floor of the orbit.

- The palatine bone articulates with the sphenoid bone pterygoid processes and with the maxillae.

Inferior Nasal Conchae

- The *inferior nasal conchae* form part of the lower one-third of the wall of the nasal cavity.

- The conchae articulate with both the ethmoid and lacrimal bones.

Vomer

- The *vomer* forms the bony portion of the nasal septum.

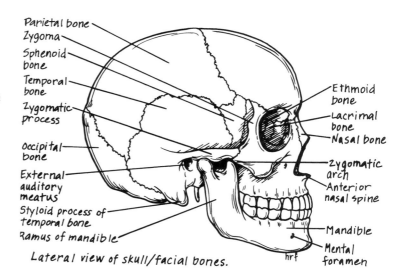

Lateral view of skull/facial bones.

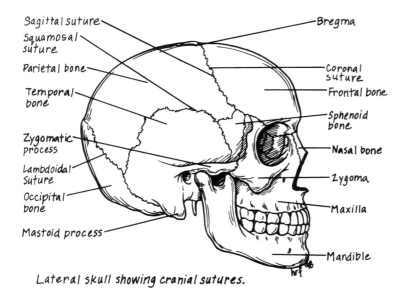

Lateral skull showing cranial sutures.

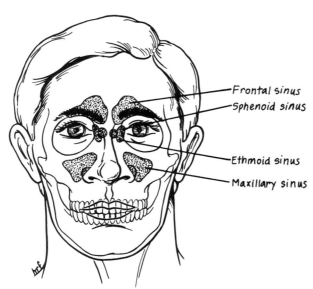

Frontal view of skull demonstrating location of paranasal sinuses.

Summary: Sutures of the Cranium

- Four major sutures are formed by the articulations of the cranial bones.

  The *coronal suture* is formed by the articulation of the frontal and two parietal bones.

  The *sagittal suture* is formed by the articulation of the two parietal bones.

  The *lambdoidal suture* is formed by articulation of the occipital and parietal bones.

  The *squamosal suture* is formed by the articulation of the parietal, temporal, and sphenoid bones.

Summary: Paranasal Sinuses

- There are four pairs of paranasal sinuses:

  Frontal frontal bone
  Ethmoid ethmoid bone
  Sphenoid sphenoid bone
  Maxillary maxillae bones.

Hyoid Bone

- The hyoid bone is a small, U-shaped bone resting at the base of the tongue. It is held in place by ligaments. The hyoid bone serves as an attachment for muscles in the throat and tongue.

PATHOPHYSIOLOGIC TERMINOLOGY ASSOCIATED WITH THE AXIAL SKELETON

Cleft palate failure of the palatine portions of the maxillae to fully unite to form the hard palate during the development of the skeleton

Herniated nucleus purposes protrusion of the disk located between two vertebrae following herniation; may place pressure on spinal nerves or the spinal cord itself.

Kyphosis an abnormality in or exaggeration of the thoracic curve causing a "humpback" appearance

Lordosis an abnormality in or exaggeration of the lumbar curve causing a "swayback" appearance

Mastoiditis an inflammation of the mastoid portion of the temporal bone

Scoliosis a lateral curvature of the vertebral column producing an S-shaped curve

Sinusitis an inflammation of the membranes of one or more of the paranasal sinuses

Spina bifida a congenital disorder in which the laminae do not unite posteriorly.

Chapter 4 Practice Questions

1. Pairs of ribs that articulate directly with the sternum via costal cartilage are known as

   a. the rib cage.
   b. true ribs.
   c. false ribs.
   d. floating ribs.

2. The upper seven pairs of ribs articulate posteriorly with _____ and anteriorly with _____.

   a. the scapula, the clavicle
   b. the scapula, the sternum
   c. a thoracic vertebra, the sternum
   d. a thoracic vertebra, costal cartilage

3. The most superior portion of the sternum is the

   a. gladiolus.
   b. body.
   c. xiphoid.
   d. manubrium.

4. Anatomically, the xiphoid lies at the level of the _____ when the body is in the erect position.

   a. eighth thoracic vertebra
   b. third thoracic vertebra
   c. tenth thoracic vertebra
   d. twelfth thoracic vertebra

5. Uniquely characteristic of the cervical vertebrae is (are) the

   a. rib facet.
   b. absence of a vertebral body.
   c. intervertebral foramina.
   d. transverse foramina.

6. The odontoid is part of which vertebral column group?

   a. cervical
   b. thoracic
   c. lumbar
   d. sacrum

7. The only vertebra with no body is the

   a. first cervical vertebra.
   b. second cervical vertebra.
   c. seventh cervical prominens.
   d. first thoracic vertebra.

8. The intervertebral foramina of the cervical vertebrae form a _____ angle from the midsagittal plane anteriorly.
   a. 35-degree
   b. 45-degree
   c. 70-degree
   d. 90-degree

9. Uniquely characteristic of the thoracic vertebrae is the presence of
   a. the thoracic prominens.
   b. a shortened spinous process.
   c. articular facets for the clavicles.
   d. articular facets for the ribs.

10. To demonstrate the apophyseal joints of the thoracic vertebrae, the body must be rotated _____ from the midsagittal plane.
    a. 35 degrees
    b. 45 degrees
    c. 70 degrees
    d. 90 degrees

11. To demonstrate the apophyseal joints of the lower lumbar, the body must be turned approximately _____ from the midsagittal plane.
    a. 35 degrees
    b. 45 degrees
    c. 70 degrees
    d. 90 degrees

12. Which of the following regions of the vertebral column serve as the posterior wall for the pelvic basin?
    a. the lumbar vertebrae
    b. the sacrum and the lumbar vertebrae
    c. the coccyx and the lumbar vertebrae
    d. the sacrum and the coccyx

13. The natural curve of the thoracic vertebrae is
    a. convex forward.
    b. concave forward.
    c. S-shaped.
    d. straight with a slight S-shape.

14. Which of the following groups of bones represent the cranial bones?
    a. frontal, maxillae, palatine, sphenoid, temporal, and occipital
    b. frontal, temporal, ethmoid, parietal, occipital, and maxillae
    c. frontal, parietal, sphenoid, temporal, occipital, and ethmoid
    d. frontal, parietal, maxillae, ethmoid, temporal, and occipital

15. The slight prominence located between the superciliary arches on the frontal bone is the
    a. supraorbital foramen.
    b. supraorbital margin.
    c. squamous portion.
    d. glabella.

16. **Which of the following groups make up the cranial bones containing the paranasal sinuses?**
    a. frontal, maxillae, ethmoid, and nasal
    b. frontal, ethmoid, sphenoid, and temporal
    c. frontal, ethmoid, and sphenoid
    d. frontal, ethmoid, and maxillae

17. **Which of the following sets of bones articulate to form the sagittal suture?**
    a. right and left parietals
    b. sphenoid and frontal
    c. temporal and parietals
    d. parietals and occipital

18. **The sella turcica is located on which of the following bones?**
    a. frontal
    b. ethmoid
    c. sphenoid
    d. temporal

19. **The organs for hearing and equilibrium are located in which of the following cranial bones?**
    a. frontal
    b. occipital
    c. temporal
    d. sphenoid

20. **The opening through which the optic nerve is connected with the brain is called the _____ and is located on the _____ cranial bone.**
    a. superior orbital fissure, frontal
    b. foramen rotundum, temporal
    c. anterior clinoid process, sphenoid
    d. optic foramen, sphenoid

21. **The mastoid process is part of the _____ bone.**
    a. frontal
    b. occipital
    c. temporal
    d. sphenoid

22. **Which of the facial bones forms the cheek?**
    a. maxilla
    b. zygoma
    c. palatine
    d. mandible

23. **At birth, the areas where cranial bones are joined together by fibrous membranes because bone tissue has not yet formed are called**
    a. orbital fissures.
    b. supraorbital fissures.
    c. fontanelles.
    d. sutures.

24. **A congenital disorder of the vertebrae in which the laminae do not unite is called**

    a. kordosis.
    b. kyphosis.
    c. scoliosis.
    d. spina bifida.

25. **Which of the facial bones contains one pair of paranasal sinuses?**

    a. mandible
    b. maxillae
    c. palatine
    d. ethmoid

The Muscular System

- The *muscular system* is made up of specialized organs that contract, causing *movement* of body parts.

- When a muscle contracts, it becomes shorter, pulling on parts that are attached and causing movement.

FUNCTIONS OF THE MUSCULAR SYSTEM

- Muscles help *maintain posture* by sustaining contraction and resisting motion.

- The gastrointestinal tract *moves food* and digested materials by muscle contractions.

- The heart is made of cardiac muscle tissue and *pumps blood* throughout the body.

- Other *body fluids* such as lymph and urine are *moved by muscles*.

- The muscular system also functions in *maintaining body heat and temperature*.

BASIC TYPES OF MUSCLE TISSUE

- There are three basic types of muscle tissue: *skeletal muscle* tissue, *smooth muscle* tissue, and *cardiac muscle* tissue.

Skeletal Muscle Tissue

- The muscles of the skeleton are covered and separated by layers of connective tissue called *fascia*.

- The fibrous connective tissue from the fascia may extend beyond the muscle to form a tendon.

- *Tendons* attach muscle to bone.

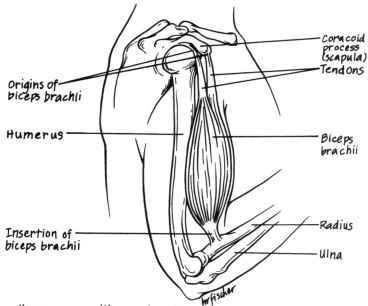

Upper arm with muscle attachments (origins and insertion).

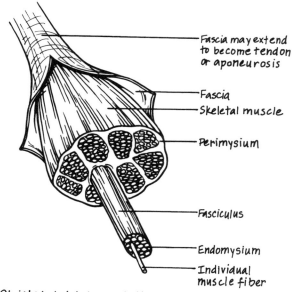

Striated skeletal muscle tissue covered by fascia.

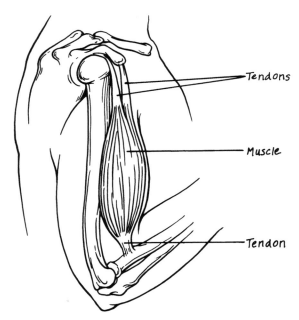

Tendons

Muscle

Tendon

Tendons attach muscle to bone.

- The fibrous connective tissue covering skeletal muscle may also extend as flat tissue that attaches one muscle to another. This flat, fibrous tissue is called an *aponeurosis.*

- The cells of muscle tissue are *elongated* and *striated* in appearance.

- Muscle cells have *cytoplasmic organelles* similar to those of a typical cell, which function to provide energy for muscle contraction.

- Muscle *cell fibers* are grouped together, however, each fiber acts as an individual unit during contraction.

- Muscles contract in response to messages received from the nervous system. When a nerve impulse is received, a nerve fiber secretes a neurotransmitter, resulting in contraction of the muscle fiber.

- A *motor unit* of contraction consists of one neuron and the muscle fibers it serves.

- When contraction occurs, all muscle cell fibers in the motor unit work together.

- The energy source for muscle contraction is *adenosine triphosphate* (ATP), an energy-carrying substance formed by cellular metabolism.

- When muscle fibers contract, *aerobic respiration*, which requires oxygen, takes place.

- During strenuous or vigorous exercise an *oxygen deficiency* may develop, resulting in an accumulation of lactic acid.

- Over a period of several hours the oxygen debt may be satisfied, which is necessary for the conversion of lactic acid to glucose, a slow process. In this way ATP that can be used for further contractions is restored.

- *Muscle fatigue* may occur, after which the muscle can no longer contract. At this point, too much lactic acid has accumulated for contraction to occur.

- Muscles not used suffer from *atrophy* and are shorter and smaller in size.

- Muscles are attached to bones by tendons. The attachment of the immovable end of the muscle is called the *origin*.

- The attachment of the movable end of the muscle is called the *insertion*.

Significant Skeletal Muscles for Radiographers

- The following muscles move the upper extremities:

  Deltoid abducts humerus, extends and flexes
  Supraspinatus abducts upper arm
  Infraspinatus rotates arm
  Biceps brachii flexes and rotates forearm
  Triceps brachii extends forearm
  Supinator rotates forearm laterally
  Pronator quadratus rotates forearm medially.

- The following muscles move the lower extremities:

  Psoas major flexes thigh
  Gluteus maximus extends the leg at the hip
  Hamstring group flexes leg at the knee
  Quadriceps group extends leg at the knee.

- The following muscles of the abdominal wall compress the contents of the abdomen and hold the abdomen in:

  External and internal obliques
  Transversus abdominis
  Rectus abdominis.

- The fibrous connective tissue that provides a longitudinal covering of the anterior abdomen is the *linea alba*.

- Muscles of the shoulder girdle are the following:

  Trapezius flexes arm, rotates and raises the scapula
  Pectoralis minor raises the ribs.

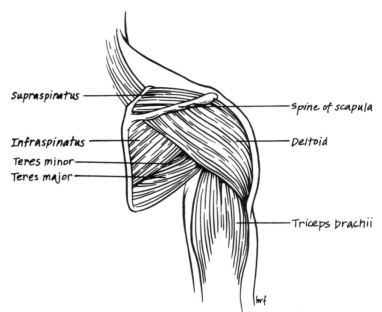

Muscle structure for upper arm (posterior aspect).

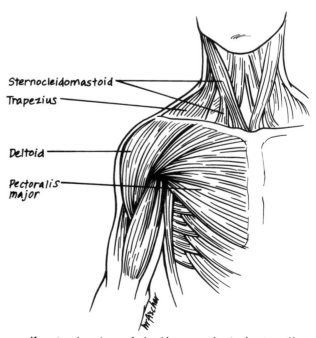

Muscle structure of shoulder area (anterior aspect).

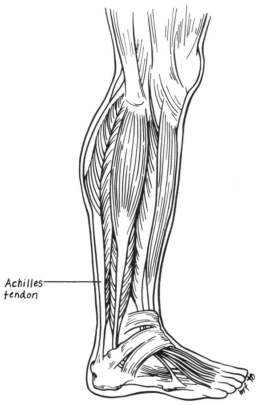

Achilles tendon

Muscles of the lower leg showing achilles tendon attachment.

- Other muscles and tendons are the following:

  Sternocleidomastoid moves the head from side to side and lowers it to the chest
  Sphincter urethrae controls the opening and closing of the urethra
  Achilles tendon attaches the posterior muscle of the lower leg to the heel bone.

Smooth Muscles

- Smooth muscles have less distinct contractions which occur in wavelike movements. This movement is called *peristalsis*.

- Smooth muscles move fluid through vessels and food through the gastrointestinal tract.

Cardiac Muscle

- The heart is made of cardiac muscle and serves as a pump to move blood throughout the body. (The structure and function of the heart muscle will be reviewed along with the cardiovascular system in Chapter 10.)

PATHOPHYSIOLOGIC TERMINOLOGY OF THE MUSCULAR SYSTEM

Muscular atrophy a decrease in size and a weakening of a muscle generally related to a lack of use
Muscular dystrophy a disorder that causes the muscles of the body to gradually degenerate
Myasthenia gravis an autoimmune disorder that gradually causes the muscles to become weakened and eventually unable to contract
Myoma a tumor in muscle tissue
Myositis an inflammation of muscle fibers
Myospasm a muscle spasm
Tendinitis an inflammation of a tendon
Tenosynovitis an inflammation of the tendons and synovial membrane around a joint

Chapter 5 Practice Questions

1. **Which of the following is not a function of the muscular system?**
   a. coordination of other systems
   b. movement of body parts
   c. maintaining posture
   d. pumping blood through the body

2. The muscles of the skeletal system are separated by layers of a type of connective tissue called

   a. organelles.
   b. cell fibers.
   c. aponeurosis.
   d. fascia.

3. One muscle is connected to another muscle by fibrous connective tissue called

   a. cell fibers.
   b. aponeurosis.
   c. fascia.
   d. ATP.

4. One neuron and the group of muscle fibers it serves are called a (an)

   a. tendon.
   b. aponeurosis.
   c. motor unit.
   d. muscle fiber unit.

5. The energy source for muscle contraction is an energy-carrying substance formed by cellular metabolism called

   a. oxygen respiration.
   b. ATP.
   c. oxygen deficiency.
   d. aerobic respiration.

6. During strenuous exercise the accumulation of lactic acid may become excessive, causing the muscle fibers to be unable to contract. This is called

   a. muscle fatigue.
   b. tetany.
   c. muscle fibrillation.
   d. muscle tonus.

7. Muscles are attached to bones by fibrous connective tissue called

   a. fascia.
   b. aponeurosis.
   c. tendons.
   d. ligaments.

8. The attachment of the movable end of a muscle is called the

   a. origin.
   b. insertion.
   c. tendon origin.
   d. motor unit attachment.

9. Which of the following muscles flexes the leg at the knee?

   a. biceps brachii group
   b. hamstring group
   c. gluteus maximus
   d. quadriceps group

10. The fibrous connective tissue providing longitudinal covering of the anterior abdominal structures is (are) the
    a. transversus abdominis.
    b. rectus abdominis.
    c. external and internal obliques.
    d. linea alba.

10. Peristalsis is a wavelike movement of the structures of the alimentary canal. This movement is produced by which type of muscle group?
    a. skeletal muscle
    b. smooth muscle
    c. striated muscle
    d. cardiac muscle

11. A decrease in the size and length of a muscle related to lack of use is called
    a. dystrophy.
    b. fatigue.
    c. atrophy.
    d. myoma.

12. An inflammation of tendons and synovial membrane around a joint is called
    a. tenosynovitis.
    b. tendinitis.
    c. synovitis.
    d. myositis.

The Nervous System

- The *nervous system* serves as the center for *coordination* and *integration* of all body systems. Coordination is essential for maintenance of the internal environment or *homeostasis*.

- The nervous system is divided into two sections: the central nervous system and the peripheral nervous system.

- The organs of the *central nervous system* are the *brain* and the *spinal cord*.

- The organs of the *peripheral nervous system* are the *nerves* connecting the more distant parts of the body to the central nervous system.

FUNCTIONS OF THE NERVOUS SYSTEM

- The nervous system *receives information*, detecting any changes in the body such as in temperature, oxygen levels, and body fluids, and *sends information* to body systems to make any needed adjustments.

- The nervous system is able to *conduct* nerve impulses in response to any need for maintaining homeostasis.

- Nerve impulses result in body movement, hormone secretions, etc.

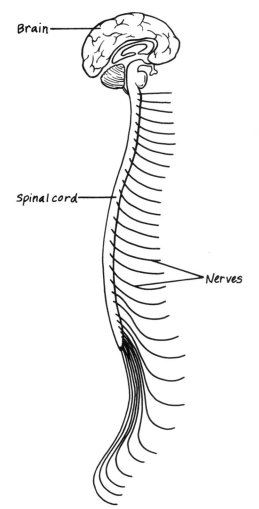

The central nervous system (brain and spinal cord) with nerves branching from spinal cord.

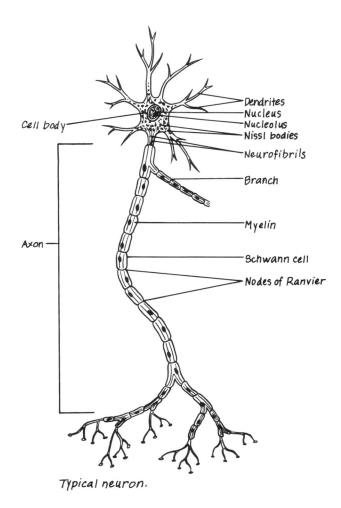

Typical neuron.

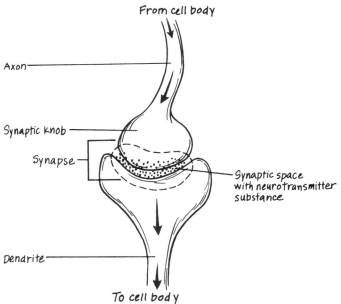

Synapse with neurotransmitter diffusing across the space between axon of one neuron to the dendrite of another neuron during nerve impulse conduction.

TISSUE STRUCTURE

- The tissue of the nervous system is composed of *neurons* and supporting tissue called *neuroglia cells*.

- Neurons may have different shapes based on their function, which is *conducting nerve impulses*.

- Neurons have a *cell body* which can be round or star-shaped. The cell body has a *nucleus* enclosed by a *nuclear membrane*.

- The nuclear membrane is surrounded by *cytoplasm* and enclosed by an outer *cell membrane*.

- The cytoplasm has *organelles* that perform specific metabolic functions and long fibrous threads called *neurofibrils*.

- The fibrous threads are continuous with extensions from the body of the cell called dendrites and axons.

- Neurons may have multiple *dendrites*, which are short extensions coming from the cell body. They have many branches and attach to sensory neurons or sensory receptors.

- Dendrites serve to conduct impulses to the cell body.

- Neurons have only one *axon* extending from the cell body.

- The axon is thicker than a dendrite and may have only one branch present on its long fiber.

- On the end of the axon most distant from the cell body are multiple branches which make contact with a receptor.

- At the very tip of the axon is the *synaptic knob*. This small, bulbous knob secretes a *neurotransmitter* which aids in the conduction of nerve impulses.

- The axon carries nerve impulses away from the cell body.

- Located between the synaptic knob and the dendrite of another neuron is the *synapse*. The synapse is a small gap or space between the two structures. The neurotransmitter aids in moving the impulse from one neuron to another.

- The larger axons are covered by tissue called *neuroglial cells.* More specifically, they are *Schwann cells* containing *myelin,* a fat-protein substance.

- *Myelinated nerve fibers* are present throughout the nervous system. These fibers appear white and therefore are called *white matter.*

- *Unmyelinated nerve fibers* appear gray and are known as *gray matter,* which is also found throughout the nervous system.

- Neuroglial cells are found in nerve tissue where they provide support for neurons and fill space. These cells are capable of *producing myelin* and carrying out *phagocytosis.*

- There are four type of neuroglial cells: astrocytes, microglia, oligodendrocytes, and ependyma.

- *Astrocytes* are located throughout nerve tissue and around blood vessels.

- *Microglia* are found throughout the nervous system and function as a cleaning system involved in phagocytosis and removal of cell debris.

- *Oligodendrocytes* are found primarily along nerve fibers and function in the production of myelin within the spinal cord and brain. They are not able to produce myelin in the peripheral nervous system.

- *Ependyma* lines the ventricles and covers specialized parts of the brain.

- Neurons are classified as multipolar, bipolar, or unipolar.

- *Multipolar neurons* have many fibers extending from the cell body, but with only one serving as the axon.

- Neurons with cell bodies that lie within the brain and spinal cord are known as multipolar neurons.

- *Bipolar neurons* have only two nerve fibers coming from the cell body. One serves as the dendrite, and the other as the axon.

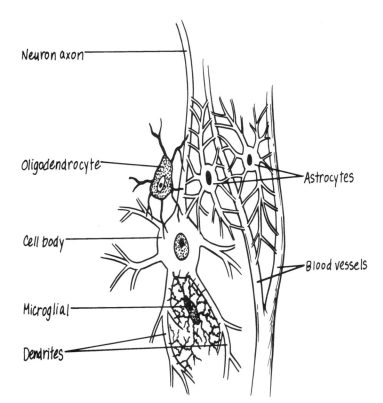

Neuroglial cells (microglial, oligodendrocyte, astrocyte) fill-in space between neurons and blood vessels.

- *Unipolar neurons* have a single fiber coming from the cell body. The single fiber branches, with one branch serving as the dendrite and the other serving as the axon.

- In unipolar neurons, the dendrite is connected with the peripheral part of the body, and the branch serving as the axon enters the brain or spinal cord.

- The cell bodies of unipolar neurons are called *ganglia* and are grouped together outside the brain and spinal cord.

- A neuron may be a sensory (afferent) neuron, a motor (efferent) neuron, or an interneuron (sometimes called an association neuron).

- *Sensory neurons* carry impulses from the periphery to the brain and spinal cord.

- *Motor neurons* carry impulses from the brain and spinal cord to other parts of the body.

- *Interneurons* lie within the brain and spinal cord and serve as connecting neurons that transmit impulses from one part of the brain or spinal cord to another part of the brain or spinal cord.

NERVE IMPULSES

- The transmission of nerve impulses is similar to the transmission of electricity. *Ions* move back and forth along the neuron nerve fiber.

- The cell membrane is *polarized* by an unequal distribution of ions on each side.

- The cell membrane is *permeable,* and certain substances can move through the membrane.

- *Potassium ions* are able to move freely back and forth across the membrane.

- *Sodium ions* are also present but do not move across the membrane as easily.

- At a normal *resting potential,* neurons have a greater concentration of potassium ions inside the membrane and sodium ions outside the membrane.

- On the inside of the membrane there is a high concentration of negative ions, and on the outside, a high concentration of positive ions.

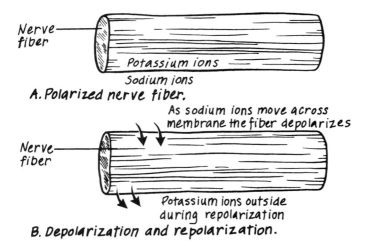

Nerve fiber

Potassium ions

Sodium ions

A. Polarized nerve fiber.

As sodium ions move across membrane the fiber depolarizes

Nerve fiber

Potassium ions outside during repolarization

B. Depolarization and repolarization.

- As *depolarization* occurs, the sodium ions move to the inside of the membrane and the potassium ions move to the outside of the membrane. As this action takes place along the nerve fiber, a nerve impulse is transmitted.

- When the fiber membrane *repolarizes*, the resting potential is reestablished.

- Myelinated nerve fibers conduct impulses much more rapidly than unmyelinated fibers.

- Nerve impulses travel first along the dendrite to the cell body and from there along the axon.

- As the impulse travels along the axon to the reach the synaptic knob, it triggers the release of the neurotransmitter (a chemical substance that varies throughout the nervous system).

- The neurotransmitter moves across the synapse, initiating an impulse in the dendrite of the connecting neuron or a response in a sensory receptor.

- The *pathway* of impulses is a *reflex arc* which normally involves a sensory neuron, an interneuron, and a motor neuron.

- *Reflexes* are reactions of the nervous system to changes in the internal or external environment or as a response to a stimulus.

CENTRAL NERVOUS SYSTEM

- The *central nervous system* includes the *brain* and the *spinal cord,* which are covered by a membrane called the *meninges.*

- The meninges have three layers: dura mater, arachnoid, and pia mater.

- The outermost layer is the *dura mater.* It is made of fibrous connective tissue and contains many blood vessels and nerves.

- The middle layer is the *arachnoid mater;* it is thinner than the dura mater and has no blood vessels.

- The innermost layer is the *pia mater* which is separated from the arachnoid mater by the *subarachnoid space.* The subarachnoid space contains *cerebrospinal fluid.*

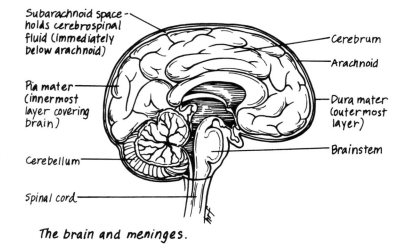

The brain and meninges.

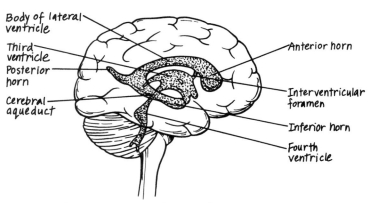

Body of lateral ventricle
Third ventricle
Posterior horn
Cerebral aqueduct
Anterior horn
Interventricular foramen
Inferior horn
Fourth ventricle

Fluid-filled ventricles of the brain.

Brain

- There are three major sections of the *brain.* The two large hemispheres are the *cerebrum,* and the most posterior is the smaller *cerebellum.* Lying in the middle and resting against the floor of the cranial cavity is the *brainstem.*

- The *cerebrum* fills most of the anterior cranial cavity. It has two hemispheres connected by a group of nerve fibers called the *corpus callosum.*

- The two hemispheres are separated by coverings of dura mater.

- The brain has many folds and ridges on the surface called *gyri* or *convolutions.*

- The ridges of the brain surface are separated by shallow and deep grooves. A shallow groove is called a *sulcus,* and a deep groove is called a *fissure.*

- The cerebrum is divided into sections each of which is named for the bone against which it lies. The sections are the *frontal lobes, temporal lobes, parietal lobes,* and *occipital lobes.*

- Located within the cerebrum are three of the four ventricles of the brain. A *ventricle* is a cavity located in the brain that contains cerebrospinal fluid.

- The two large *lateral ventricles* are located in the cerebrum and occupy much of the frontal, temporal, parietal, and occipital lobes.

- Just below the corpus callosum in the mid-sagittal plane is the *third ventricle.*

- The cerebrum is covered by the outer *cerebral cortex,* which is a thin layer of *gray matter.*

- Most motor and sensory areas are found in the cerebrum along with interpretative centers.

- The *cerebellum* is a large mass of brain tissue located inferior to the occipital lobes of the cerebrum.

- The cerebellum has two hemispheres separated by the dura mater. These two hemispheres are connected by the *vermis.*

- The cerebellum is covered with gray matter which is known as the *cerebellar cortex.*

- The cerebellum functions as a reflex center and coordinates movement of skeletal muscles; it also coordinates muscle contraction to maintain posture.

- The *brainstem* is a bundle of nerve tissue connecting the spinal cord to the cerebrum.

- The tissue in the brainstem contains nerve fibers and gray mater.

- The brainstem has four sections: the diencephalon, midbrain, pons, and medulla oblongata.

- The *diencephalon* lies in the midsagittal region just above the midbrain and is encircled by the third ventricle of the brain.

- The diencephalon contains the *thalamus*, which serves as a relay center, the *hypothalamus,* which plays a major role in homeostasis, the *limbic system,* which is the center of emotions and expression, and the *pineal gland.*

- The *fourth ventricle* of the brain is located in the brainstem. It is anterior to the cerebellum and posterior to the pons. The fourth ventricle is connected to the third ventricle superiorly by a small duct called the *cerebral aqueduct.*

- The *midbrain* is a group of myelinated fibers that connect the brain and the spinal cord.

- The *pons* consists primarily of nerve fibers that serve to separate the midbrain from the medulla oblongata.

- The *medulla oblongata* is the enlarged portion of the spinal cord connecting the spinal cord and the rest of the brainstem. It rests in and above the *foramen magnum* of the occipital bone.

- The medulla oblongata functions as a control center regulating the heart rate and dilation and constriction of blood vessels, and as a respiratory center controlling the rate of breathing.

- There are 12 pairs of *cranial nerves* rising from several locations in the brain.

- The first pair of cranial nerves come from the cerebrum, and the remaining 11 pairs arise from the brainstem.

- The 12 cranial nerves control vision, eye movement, smell, facial movements, swallowing, hearing, equilibrium, movement of the tongue, and other movements of the head.

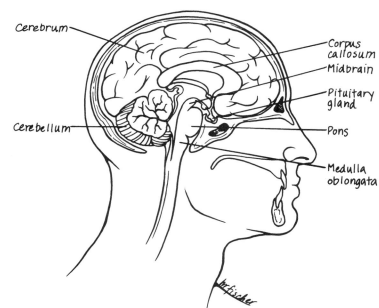

Brainstem and cerebellum in relationship to the cerebrum.

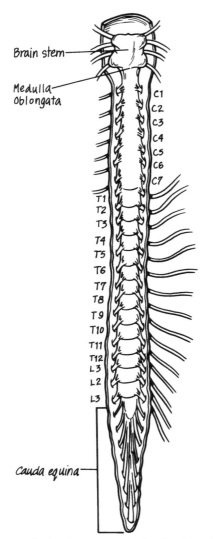

Brain stem

Medulla
Oblongata

C1
C2
C3
C4
C5
C6
C7

T1
T2
T3
T4
T5
T6
T7
T8
T9
T10
T11
T12
L3
L2
L3

Cauda equina

Anterior aspect of spinal cord.

Spinal Cord

- The *spinal cord* is the long bundle of nerve tissue extending from the brain at the level of the foramen magnum to about L2.

- In the vertebral canal, the spinal cord is surrounded and protected by the bones of the vertebral column. The spinal cord ends at approximately L1 or L2. Extending beyond this point is a bundle of nerve fibers called the *cauda equina.*

- There are 31 pairs of *spinal nerves* which branch from the spinal cord and exit the vertebral canal through the intervertebral foramen.

- The function of the spinal cord is to conduct impulses from peripheral parts of the body to the brain and back. In addition, it functions as a reflex center.

AUTONOMIC NERVOUS SYSTEM

- The *autonomic nervous system* is embedded within the nervous system and functions independently of conscious control.

- The main control centers of the autonomic nervous system are the *hypothalamus* and the *medulla oblongata.*

- There are two divisions of the autonomic nervous system: the sympathetic and the parasympathetic.

- The *sympathetic system* assists the body in responding to stressful and emergency conditions.

- The *parasympathetic system* maintains control of the body under normal or ordinary conditions.

- The autonomic nervous system plays a significant role in the regulation of peristalsis of smooth muscles, secretion from glands, the cardiac rate, breathing, body temperature, and blood pressure.

- The autonomic nervous systems responds when the body is under emotional and physical stress.

PATHOPHYSIOLOGIC TERMINOLOGY ASSOCIATED WITH THE NERVOUS SYSTEM

Alzheimer's disease degeneration of the brain causing atrophy and eventually death

Amyotrophic lateral sclerosis (Lou Gehrig's disease) a chronic progressive disease of the nervous system which occurs later in life; characterized by muscle atrophy and hardening of areas of the spinal cord

Aphasia the inability to write or speak due to brain damage

Arnold-Chiari syndrome congenital malformation of the cerebellum with displacement of the fourth ventricle

Astrocytoma a tumor originating in astrocyte cells.

Ataxia a disorder of the nervous system causing a loss of muscular coordination

Bell's palsy a palsy causing weakness of the peripheral facial nerve

Cardiovascular accident (CVA) Bleeding in the brain caused by a rupture of an artery; if bleeding is excessive death will result

Cephalocele protrusion of the brain due to a defect in a cranial bone

Cerebral hemorrhage bleeding into the cerebrum as a result of trauma or rupture of an artery

Cerebral palsy loss of control and coordination of muscle movement due to brain damage

Comatose a condition in which one is unable to respond to a stimulus

Dementia mental deterioration caused by an organic disease of the brain

Encephalitis an inflammation of the brain; can be any one of a variety of types

Encephalomyelitis an inflammation of the brain and spinal cord

Epidural hematoma a collection of blood outside the dura mater

Epilepsy a disorder of the nervous system associated with frequent convulsions that may be of the grand mal or petit mal type; convulsions occur as a result of disturbances of brain impulses

Glioblastoma multiforme a malignant tumor of the cerebrum

Guillain-Barré syndrome an infectious neurologic condition causing weakness, pain, and paralysis (sometimes only temporary), usually caused by a virus

Hemiplegia paralysis on one side of the body.

Huntington's chorea a hereditary progressive disease of the nervous system occurring after 30 years of age and resulting in degeneration of the brain, irritability, and personality change

Hydrocephalus a congenital condition characterized by an enlarged ventricle, an enlarged cranium, and a thin cerebral cortex

Intracranial hemorrhage leakage of blood within the cranial cavity causing a hematoma

Medulloblastoma a malignant tumor of the cerebellum

Meningioma a benign tumor of the arachnoid tissue

Meningitis an inflammation of the meninges of the brain and spinal cord that is usually of viral or bacterial origin

Meningocele herniation of the meninges through a defect in the bone

Microcephalus a small head

Multiple sclerosis a nervous system disorder resulting in demyelination of nerve tissue in the brain and the spinal cord; usually appears early in adult life with intermittent progression leading to paralysis, ataxia, lack of muscle coordination, and speech disturbances

Narcolepsy the uncontrolled urge to sleep

Neuritis an inflammation of nerves

Neuroblastoma a malignant tumor composed primarily of neuroblasts

Neurofibroma a tumor of peripheral nerve cells caused by the proliferation of Schwann cells

Paralysis a loss of motor function

Paraplegia paralysis of the lower torso and the lower extremities

Parkinson's disease a disease occurring later in life characterized by tremor and muscle rigidity

Poliomyelitis viral infection and inflammation of the gray matter of the spinal cord caused by poliovirus

Polyneuritis inflammation of a large number of nerves at one time

Subarachnoid hemorrhage leakage of blood into the subarachnoid space; cerebrospinal fluid normally shows the presence of red blood cells

Subdural hematoma leakage of blood into the space between the dura mater and the arachnoid

Syncope loss of consciousness for a short period due to a decrease in blood flow to the cerebrum; can result from a drop in blood pressure

Chapter 6 Practice Questions

1. Which of the following is not a function of the nervous system?
   a. secretion of fluids
   b. conduction of nerve impulses
   c. coordination of body systems
   d. receiving and sending of information from one part of the body to another

2. The basic nerve cell for coĭucting nerve impulses is the
   a. astrocyte.
   b. myelin.
   c. neuron.
   d. oligodendrocyte.

3. Neurons with cell bodies that lie within the brain and spinal cord are called
   a. bipolar neurons.
   b. unipolar.
   c. multipolar.
   d. ependymal.

4. Neurons that carry impulses from the brain and spinal cord to other parts of the body are known as
   a. interneurons.
   b. association neurons.
   c. sensory neurons.
   d. motor neurons.

5. Which of the following is the outermost layer of the meninges?
   a. corpus callosum
   b. arachnoid
   c. dura mater
   d. pia mater

6. Cerebrospinal fluid circulates in the
   a. extradural space.
   b. epidural space.
   c. subdural space.
   d. subarachnoid space.

7. Fluid-filled cavities located in the cerebrum and brainstem are called
   a. gyri.
   b. convolutions.
   c. fissures.
   d. ventricles.

8. The part of the brainstem that encircles the third ventricle is known as the
   a. diencephalon.
   b. midbrain.
   c. pons.
   d. medulla oblongata.

9. There are _____ pairs of spinal nerves.
   a. 12
   b. 24
   c. 31
   d. 33

10. Herniation of the meninges through a defect in the bone is called
    a. encephalitis.
    b. an epidural hematoma.
    c. Guillain-Barré syndrome.
    d. a meningocele.

The Endocrine System

- The endocrine system and the nervous system coordinate and integrate the internal environment to maintain homeostasis. The *nervous system* coordinates and integrates systems via *nerve impulses*, and the *endocrine system* by the release of *hormones*.

- The endocrine system is composed of tissue and organs located throughout the body that secrete hormones.

- Hormone secretions can stimulate another endocrine gland to secrete its hormone or to secrete a hormone that directly initiates an action within the body.

- Hormone secretions are very concentrated and are required in very small amounts.

- The release of hormones by the endocrine glands is regulated by a *negative feedback* process. When the amount of hormone secretion falls below the amount required by the body, a gland is stimulated to produce more. The release of some hormones is through nerve impulse.

- The endocrine glands are the pituitary, pineal, thyroid, parathyroid, thymus, digestive, adrenal, pancreas, and reproductive glands (ovaries and the testes).

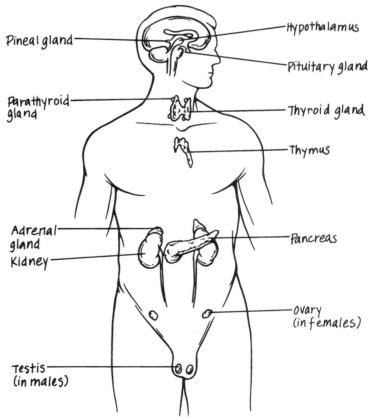

The organs of the endocrine system.

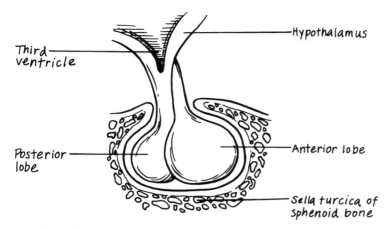

Anterior and posterior lobe of pituitary gland resting in the sella turcica of sphenoid bone.

PITUITARY GLAND

- The *pituitary gland* is called the "master" gland because it regulates most of the hormone secretions of the other endocrine glands.

- The pituitary gland lies in the *sella turcica*, which is at the base of the brain.

- The pituitary gland is attached to the hypothalamus by a stalk called the *infundibulum* and is divided into two lobes.

Anterior Lobe

- The *anterior lobe* secretes the following hormones:

    Growth hormone
    Thyroid-stimulating hormone
    Follicle-stimulating hormone
    Prolactin
    Adrenocorticotropic hormone
    Luteinizing hormone.

- *Growth hormone* (GH) stimulates the growth and reproduction of body cells.

- *Thyroid-stimulating hormone* (TSH) controls the secretion of hormones by the thyroid gland.

- *Follicle-stimulating hormone* (FSH) initiates development of the egg-producing follicles in the ovaries.

- *Prolactin*, produced by lactating women, sustains milk production following birth.

- *Adrenocorticotropic hormone* (ACTH) controls the release of specific hormones of the adrenal cortex.

- *Luteinizing hormone* (LH) controls the release of the egg from the follicle in females.

Posterior Lobe

- The *posterior lobe* of the pituitary gland secretes the following hormones:

    Antidiuretic hormone
    Oxytocin.

- *Antidiuretic hormone* (ADH) causes the kidneys to reduce water release.

- *Oxytocin* causes the walls of the uterine wall to contract and stimulates the milk-producing glands to release milk.

PINEAL GLAND

- The *pineal gland* is located in the middle of the cerebrum and is attached to the *thalamus.*

- The pineal gland is known to secrete *melatonin,* which is believed to inhibit the release of gonadotropins from the pituitary gland.

THYROID GLAND

- The *thyroid gland* is located in the anterior neck area just below the larynx.

- The following hormones are secreted by the thyroid gland:

    Triiodothyronine
    Thyroxine
    Calcitonin.

- *Triiodothyronine* is a hormone that increases the rate at which energy is released through carbohydrate and protein metabolism. It also increases nervous system activity.

- *Thyroxine* is a hormone that performs the same functions as triiodothyronine.

- *Calcitonin* lowers the levels of calcium and phosphate ions in the body.

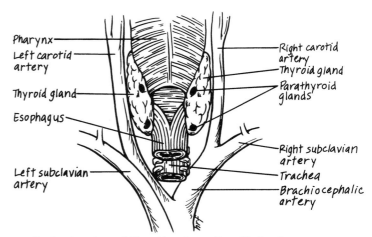

Posterior view of thyroid and parathyroid glands and associated anatomy.

PARATHYROID GLANDS

- The *parathyroid glands* are four small glands located on the posterior surface of the thyroid gland.

- The hormone secreted by the parathyroid gland is *parathyroid hormone.* This hormone serves to decrease the concentration of phosphate in the blood.

THYMUS GLAND

- The *thymus gland* is located in the chest cavity just posterior to the sternum.

- The hormone released by the thymus is thymosin, which affects the production of blood cells called *lymphocytes.*

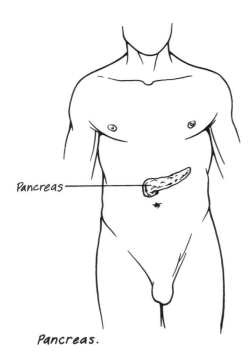

Pancreas.

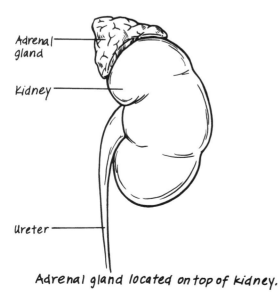

Adrenal gland located on top of kidney.

PANCREAS

- The *pancreas* is located in the upper abdominal cavity. It is a long gland that is attached by ducts opening into the proximal end of the small intestine.

- The pancreas has a *double function*. It serves as an *endocrine gland*, secreting the hormones insulin and glucagon. The pancreas also acts as an *exocrine gland* by secreting digestive juices into the digestive tract.

- The endocrine portion of the gland is a group of cells called the *islets of Langerhans*.

- The two types of cells within the islets of Langerhans are *alpha cells*, which secrete glucagon, and *beta cells*, which secrete insulin.

- The hormone *glucagon* stimulates the conversion of glycogen to glucose. This occurs by a negative feedback mechanism and maintains the blood glucose level. When needed, glucagon elevates blood sugar levels.

- *Insulin* secreted by the beta cells works to decrease blood glucose levels. It functions to facilitate the conversion of glucose to glycogen which can be stored. It also facilitates the diffusion of glucose through cell membranes to support cellular metabolism.

- A common disorder of the pancreas, *diabetes mellitus,* is characterized by an inability to produce insulin or by the production of only a minimal amount that is inadequate for glucose metabolism.

DIGESTIVE GLANDS

- The *digestive glands* are located within the lining of the stomach and small intestine.

- These glands secrete hormones that aid in digestion.

ADRENAL GLANDS

- The *adrenal glands* are "caps" resting on the top of the kidneys.

- The adrenal glands are very vascular and are separated into two sections.

- The outer thicker portion covering the surface of the gland is the *adrenal cortex.*

- The inner portion is the *adrenal medulla.* Each section secretes hormones.

- The hormones secreted by the adrenal cortex are aldosterone, cortisol, and sex hormones (androgen, estrogen, and progesterone)

- *Aldosterone* is a hormone that helps regulate the concentration of extracellular electrolytes.

- *Cortisol* facilitates the metabolism of fats, carbohydrates, and protein.

- *Sex hormones* supplement those produced by the ovaries and testes and help stimulate development of the sex organs.

REPRODUCTIVE GLANDS

- In the female the *reproductive glands* are the *ovaries,* which produce estrogen and progesterone.

- The *placenta* is also considered an endocrine gland because it produces estrogen, progesterone, and gonadotropin.

- In the male the *testes* produce testosterone.

PATHOPHYSIOLOGIC TERMINOLOGY ASSOCIATED WITH THE ENDOCRINE SYSTEM

Addison's disease a disease associated with adrenal gland insufficiency; may be accompanied by darkened skin, anemia, and general weakness, and it may be life-threatening.

Adrenal cortical carcinoma a malignant tumor of the adrenal gland

Chromophobic adenoma a benign tumor of the pituitary gland

Cretinism a permanent condition of stunted growth due to hypothyroidism in infancy

Cushing's syndrome hypersecretion of adrenocorticotropic hormone by the pituitary gland

Diabetes insipidus a disorder of the posterior lobe of the pituitary gland caused by hyposecretion of antidiuretic hormone (ADH); symptoms include excessive elimination of urine and excessive thirst

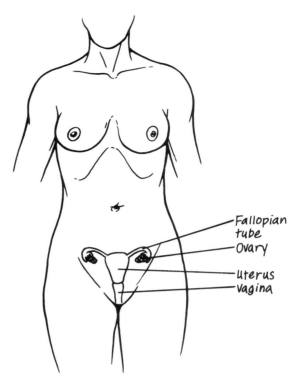

Female reproductive organs (ovaries located in abdominal cavity).

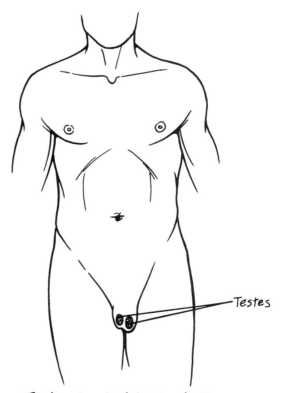

Testes located in scrotum.

Diabetes mellitus type I is caused by an insufficiency of insulin production by the beta cells of the pancreas, resulting in a deficiency of insulin which is required for cells to obtain and use glucose (also called insulin-dependent diabetes); type II is usually classified as a disease of later life characterized by high glucose levels in the blood and is usually controlled by diet, exercise, and weight loss

Dwarfism hyposecretion of growth hormone by the pituitary gland

Goiter enlargement of the thyroid gland

Hyperparathyroidism oversecretion of parathyroid hormone resulting in hypocalcemia and calcium imbalance

Hyperthyroidism hypersecretion of thyroid hormone

Hypoparathyroidism hyposecretion of the parathyroid hormone

Hypothyroidism hyposecretion of thyroid hormone

Myxedema skin dryness and intolerance of cold due to hyposecretion of thyroid hormone.

Chapter 7 Practice Questions

1. The endocrine gland known as the "master" gland is the
   a. pineal gland.
   b. pituitary gland.
   c. adrenal gland.
   d. pancreas.

2. FSH is secreted by which of the following endocrine glands?
   a. adrenal gland
   b. ovary
   c. thyroid
   d. pituitary

3. ADH functions to maintain water balance and is secreted by the
   a. anterior lobe of the pituitary gland.
   b. posterior lobe of the pituitary gland.
   c. thymus gland.
   d. adrenal gland.

4. Which of the following functions as both an endocrine and an exocrine gland?
   a. thymus
   b. parathyroid
   c. pancreas
   d. adrenals

5. The hormone required for glucose metabolism is

   a. glycogen.
   b. insulin.
   c. ADH.
   d. ACTH.

6. Cortisol facilitates the metabolism of fats, carbohydrates, and protein. It is secreted by which of the following endocrine glands?

   a. pituitary
   b. thyroid
   c. pancreas
   d. adrenal

7. Skin dryness and intolerance to cold due to hyposecretion of the thyroid gland is a symptom of

   a. Cushing's syndrome.
   b. Addison's disease.
   c. myxedema.
   d. diabetes insipidus.

8. Insufficiency of insulin production by beta cells is a characteristic of

   a. diabetes insipidus.
   b. diabetes mellitus.
   c. cretinism.
   d. goiter.

9. The process involving the release of hormones by endocrine glands is

   a. diffusion.
   b. osmosis.
   c. positive feedback.
   d. negative feedback.

10. Which of the following hormones is needed for the conversion of glycogen to glucose?

   a. glucagon
   b. glycogen
   c. insulin
   d. oxytocin

The Sensory System

- The body has *special senses* that serve as receptors for gathering information about what is going on outside the body as well as inside.

- These *special receptors* are able to detect even minute changes in the environment.

- The special senses are *hearing* and *equilibrium, vision, taste,* and *smell.* They function as an alarm system, letting the organism know when it is in danger.

- The *somatic senses* are found throughout the body, allowing the body to experience *touch, pressure, pain,* and *temperature.*

- All the sense organs are connected to the *nervous system.* When a sensory organ is stimulated, a nerve impulse is sent through a nerve pathway to the central nervous system where the information is processed and interpreted.

- Each sensory receptor responds only to a distinct or special change in the environment and therefore responds to only one type of stimulus.

RECEPTORS

- *Receptors* are usually classified relative to their sensitivity.

- The body has five basic groups of receptors: mechanoreceptors, photoreceptors, chemoreceptors, pain receptors, and thermoreceptors.

- A *mechanoreceptor* responds to changes in pressure and movement of fluid, for example, receptors in the ear.

- A *photoreceptor* responds to different energies given off by light, for example, receptors in the eye.

- A *chemoreceptor* responds to changes in chemical concentrations, as in the sense of smell.

- *Pain receptors* respond to tissue damage, and *thermoreceptors* respond to changes in temperature.

- Sensory impulses are interpreted by the brain as *sensations*. The brain sends the feeling or sensation back to the source of the impulse or back to where the stimulus occurred. This process is called *projection*. For example, a burn on the finger is interpreted by the brain as heat and pain, but the sensations are felt on the finger.

- Sensory *receptors adapt* with continuous stimulation. This results in a cessation of impulses being sent to the brain unless the stimulus increases in strength or in concentration.

- The sense of smell functions this way. An unpleasant odor is smelled, but the sense organ involved adapts quickly (in about 1 minute or less). In order to continue to smell the odor the concentration must be changed, which can be done by "sniffing" the odor.

HEARING AND EQUILIBRIUM

- The organ of *hearing* and *equilibrium* is the ear. The ear is divided into *external*, *middle*, and *inner* sections located in the temporal bone of the skull.

The External Ear

- The parts of the *external ear* are the *auricle* (ear lobe) and a slightly curved canal called the *external auditory meatus* (EAM). The EAM ends at the *tympanic membrane*, also known as the eardrum.

- The shape of the auricle helps sound to enter the EAM and cause the tympanic membrane to vibrate.

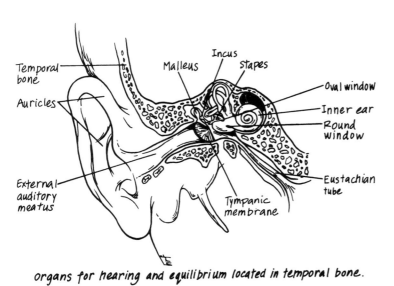

organs for hearing and equilibrium located in temporal bone.

The Middle Ear

- The *middle ear* is an air-filled cavity that begins at the tympanic membrane and contains three very tiny bones called *ossicles*, also known as the *malleus* (hammer), *incus* (anvil), and *stapes* (stirrup).

- The stapes is attached by ligaments to the *oval window* located on the vestibule of the labyrinth (inner ear).

- The ossicles vibrate as a result of movement of the tympanic membrane. The vibration is caused by sound waves entering the EAM.

- As the ossicles vibrate, the stapes stimulates movement of the fluid located in the inner ear structures, which in turn stimulates the organ of hearing located in the inner ear.

- The *middle ear cavity*, also known as the *tympanic cavity*, has an opening on the inferior surface. This opening connects the middle ear to the pharynx via a tube called the eustachian tube.

- The *eustachian tube* is an open tube that allows air pressure within the middle ear to remain stable.

Middle ear ossicles with surrounding structures.

The Inner Ear

- The *inner ear* is a *bony labyrinth* consisting of circular and coiled structures. Inside the bony structure are layers of fluid and a *membranous structure* identical in shape to the labyrinth.

- Between the bony outer layer of the labyrinth and the membranous labyrinth is a fluid called *perilymph*. Inside the membranous labyrinth is a fluid called *endolymph*.

- The three circular structures in the inner ear are called *semicircular canals* and lie at right angles to one another. The receptors for equilibrium are located in the semicircular canals. The inner coiled structure is the *cochlea*, which contains the receptors for hearing.

- Between the semicircular canals and the cochlea is the *vestibule*. The vestibule has two chambers called the *utricle* and the *saccule*, both of which function in maintaining equilibrium.

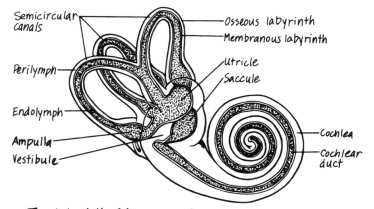

The labyrinth of inner ear with bony and membranous labyrinths.

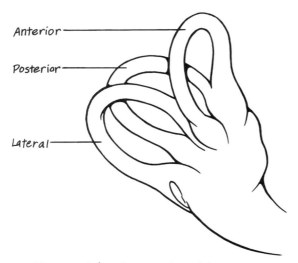

Anterior

Posterior

Lateral

The semicircular canals which contain the organs of equilibrium.

Sense of Equilibrium

- The sense of *equilibrium* involves the receptors in the utricle being stimulated by pressure from the fluid in the semicircular canals. This stimulation occurs when the head is moved forward, backward, or to the side.

- The impulse received by the equilibrium receptors is sent to the brain, which then sends impulses to the skeletal muscles, causing them to contract or relax as needed to maintain balance.

Sense of Hearing

- The organ of *hearing* that contains the receptors is the *organ of Corti* and is located in the cochlea. The organ of Corti has hairlike extensions which project outward and is covered by a very thin membrane.

- As sound is received by the external ear, the tympanic membrane vibrates, and these vibrations cause the ossicles to move. The stapes vibrates against the oval window, stimulating the fluid in the inner ear labyrinth.

- As the fluid inside the cochlea begins to move, the wavelike motion stimulates the organ of Corti by moving the hairlike projections. This results in the creation of a nerve impulse which is interpreted by the brain as sound.

SENSE OF VISION

- The organ of *vision* is the eye. Also involved in the sense of vision are the *accessory organs* of the eye: the tear ducts or sacs, extrinsic muscles, eyelids, and conjunctiva.

- The eye rests in an orbit of the skull. The *optic nerve* leaves the eye through the *optic foramen* in the sphenoid bone and connects with the brain.

- The eye is a hollow structure with three basic layers that form the walls. The *outer layer* is the fibrous tunic, the *middle layer* is the vascular tunic, and the *innermost layer* is the nervous tunic.

Posterior cavity

Sclera

Optic nerve

Optic disk

Fovea centralis

Choroid coat

Retina

Ciliary body

Suspensory ligaments

Posterior chamber

Anterior chamber

Anterior cavity

Pupil

Lens

Iris

Aqueous humor

Cornea

Lateral aspect of the eye, the organ for vision.

- On the anterior surface of the outer *or fibrous tunic* is the *cornea*. The *sclera*, also part of the fibrous tunic, continues from the cornea around the remaining part of the eye. The opening through which the optic nerve passes as it exits the eye is located on the posterior surface of the sclera.

- The cornea is transparent and permits light to enter the eye. Just posterior to the cornea is the *anterior chamber* which is filled with a fluid called *aqueous humor.*

- The middle or *vascular tunic* contains the *iris*, which is a thin, muscular structure located on the anterior surface behind the cornea and aqueous humor. The iris is the colored portion of the eye. The opening in the iris is the *pupil*. The pupil allows aqueous humor to move from the anterior chamber to the *posterior chamber.*

- Directly behind the iris is the *lens*, which is held in place by *suspended ligaments*.

- The middle tunic also contains the *ciliary body*, which functions to shorten or lengthen the lens, a process that accommodates near and far vision.

- The *choroid coat* is part of the middle tunic. It is loosely connected to the sclera and has numerous blood vessels. Pigments found in the choroid coat enable it to absorb excess light.

- The innermost or *nervous tunic* is the retina. The retina contains the photoreceptors for vision, which are distributed over its posterior and lateral surfaces.

- The *fovea centralis* is located in the center posteriorly and is seen as a small depression in the retina where vision is the sharpest. Adjacent to the fovea centralis is the optic disk. The *optic disk* is where the nerve fibers of the optic nerve come together and leave the eye. It is the location of the *blind spot*, which has no receptors.

- The visual receptors are the rods and cones. *Rods* are more sensitive to light and allow one to see in extremely low light.

- *Cones* are more active in daylight and detect color. Vision is usually sharper with stimulation of the cones, however, the rods contribute to peripheral vision.

- The light-sensitive pigment in the eye is called *rhodopsin*.

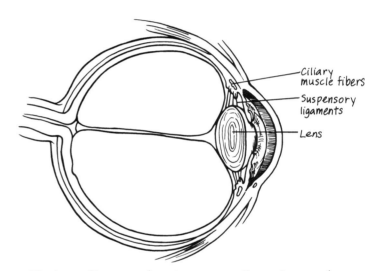

The lens, ciliary muscle and suspensory ligaments serve to accommodate for viewing close objects or far away (the ciliary fibers contract, suspensory ligaments relax and the lens becomes more convex when viewing close-up objects).

The Nature of Vision

- Light enters the eye, and the energy given off from the light stimulates the rods and cones. The sensitive pigment in the rods and cones responds with chemical changes, initiating a nerve impulse which is sent to the brain for interpretation. The sensation that results is vision with objects shown in different colors.

SENSE OF TASTE

- The organs of taste are the *taste buds,* which are mostly concentrated on the tongue but are also located on the walls and roof of the mouth.

- A taste bud is composed of epithelial cells which serve as taste receptors. Taste bud cells have openings with tiny hairs or projections protruding outward from the ends of the cells. Nerve fibers are connected to these cells and, when stimulated, provide a sensation of taste.

- Before any substance can be detected, it must be mixed with fluid secreted by the salivary glands.

- Certain locations on the tongue have cells that detect specific tastes. A *sweet taste* is detected by cells located on the anterior surface of the tongue. A *sour taste* is detected more by cells located on the lateral edges of the tongue. A *bitter taste* is detected at the back of the tongue, and a *salty taste* along the edges of the tongue.

- The sense of taste is enhanced by the sense of smell.

SENSE OF SMELL

- The organs of smell are the *olfactory cells* located in the upper part of the nasal cavity and on the nasal septum.

- The *olfactory receptors* are specialized epithelial cells with hairy knobs on their ends.

- As chemicals or gases enter the nasal cavity and mix with moisture located there, the knobs on the cells detect their presence, resulting in a nerve impulse being sent to the brain which is interpreted as smell.

- Olfactory cells are known to adapt very rapidly.

Olfactory bulb
Cribriform plate of ethmoid bone
Nasal conchae
Nasal cavity

Sense organ for smell located in upper portion of nasal cavity.

SOMATIC SENSES

- The somatic senses include touch, pressure, pain, and temperature.

- *Touch* and *pressure* receptors are located in epithelial cells found on the external surfaces of the body.

- The receptors for touch are called *Meissner corpuscles,* and the receptors for pressure are known as *Pacinian corpuscles.*

- The sense of *temperature*, or hot and cold, is felt by receptors connected to nerves located in the skin.

- Tissue damage stimulates a *pain* receptor. Pain receptors are located on the outside of the body and in organs within the body. There are no pain receptors in the brain.

PATHOPHYSIOLOGIC TERMINOLOGY ASSOCIATED WITH THE SENSORY SYSTEM

Acoustic neuroma a tumor in the internal auditory meatus arising from the acoustic nerve; without surgical intervention the tumor will spread toward the brain, wrapping around the facial and trigeminal nerves

Astigmatism a disorder of the cornea or lens resulting in images being out of focus

Blepharitis an inflammation of the eyelid

Conjunctivitis an inflammation of the conjunctiva of the eye

Dacryocystitis an inflammation of the lacrimal gland and sac

Keratitis an inflammation of the cornea

Menière's syndrome progressive deafness associated with dizziness

Optic neuritis an inflammation of the optic nerve

Otalgia an earache

Otitis media an inflammation of the middle ear

Otosclerosis formation of bony tissue around the stapes and oval window which prevents vibration and causes deafness

Tinnitus a ringing in the ears

Chapter 8 Practice Questions

1. The senses that respond to touch and pain are the
   a. special senses.
   b. special receptors.
   c. somatic senses.
   d. olfactory senses.

2. The type of receptor that responds to pressure and movement of fluid is the
   a. mechanoreceptor.
   b. photoreceptor.
   c. chemoreceptor.
   d. thermoreceptor.

3. Which part of the inner ear anatomy is the center of equilibrium?
   a. oval window
   b. round window
   c. cochlea
   d. semicircular canals

4. The middle ear cavity is separated from the external ear by the _____, and from the inner ear by the _____.
   a. stapes, oval window
   b. tympanic membrane, cochlea
   c. tympanic membrane, oval window
   d. EAM, semicircular canals

5. The bony labyrinth and membranous labyrinth are separated by the
   a. tympanic membrane.
   b. vestibule.
   c. middle ear cavity.
   d. perilymph.

6. The organ of hearing is the
   a. utricle.
   b. saccule.
   c. organ of Corti.
   d. ossicle.

7. Which of the following is not an accessory organ of the eye?
   a. pupil
   b. conjunctiva
   c. lens
   d. ciliary body

8. The layer of tissue surrounding the eye that contains the blood vessels is the
   a. outermost layer with the cornea.
   b. sclera.
   c. retina.
   d. middle layer with the choroid coat.

9. **The center of sharpest vision is the**
    a. retina.
    b. lens.
    c. fovea centralis.
    d. optic nerve.

10. **Inflammation of the eyelid is called**
    a. astigmatism.
    b. blepharitis.
    c. dacryocystitis
    d. optic neuritis.

The Digestive System

THE DIGESTIVE SYSTEM

- The organs of the *digestive system* include the *alimentary canal* and accessory glands including the *salivary glands, gallbladder, liver,* and *pancreas.*

- The function of the digestive system is to take in food and nutrients and process the food into a form that can be used by cells for metabolism and the production of energy.

- The digestive system serves as a passageway for the elimination of waste products produced by digestion.

THE ALIMENTARY CANAL

- The *alimentary canal* is a long tube, which if removed and stretched would be about 9 m (30 ft) in length. It has muscles that run circularly and longitudinally along the walls of the canal and produce peristalsis when contracted.

- The canal begins at the *mouth* and continues through the *pharynx, esophagus, stomach, small* and *large intestines, rectum,* and *anal canal,* ending at the *anus,* the muscle sphincter opening to the outside.

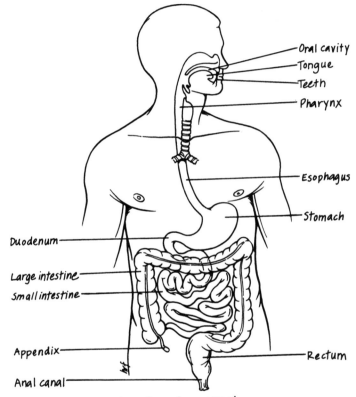

The organs of the alimentary canal.

Mucosal Lining of the Canal

- Lining the alimentary canal is a *mucous membrane* made up of epithelial cells with connective tissue underneath serving as support. The mucous membrane secretes substances needed for digestion and has special characteristics enabling it to absorb nutrients to be used for cellular metabolism.

- The mucosal folds and projections so vital for secretion and absorption may vary from organ to organ based on the specific function of the organ.

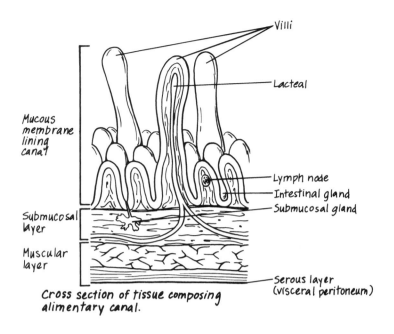

Cross section of tissue composing alimentary canal.

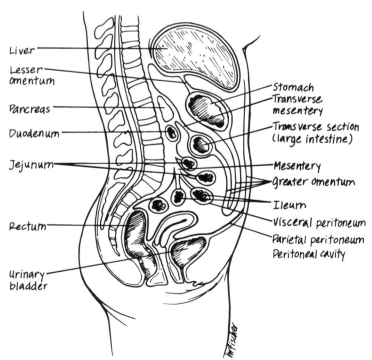

Lateral aspect of abdominal cavity shows peritoneum and its extensions in relationship to organs of alimentary canal.

- The tissue layers of the tube or alimentary canal are the mucosal, submucosal, muscular, and serous layers.

- The inner *mucosal layer* serves to protect the sublayers and has projections called *villi* which contain intestinal glands and lymph nodes. The mucosal lining *secretes digestive juices* for mixing with food to ready it for digestion and absorption. Mucosal patterns are of great importance in radiographic imaging of the gastrointestinal tract in evaluating the inner lining of the alimentary canal for ulcers or other types of lesions.

- The *submucosal layer* contains loose connective tissue heavily saturated with nerves, blood, and lymphatic vessels.

- The *muscular layer* contains the muscles that encircle the canal and longitudinal muscle fibers that work together to produce peristalsis. *Peristalsis* is the contraction of circular and longitudinal muscles along the alimentary canal by which food is moved into the stomach and intestines and waste materials or feces are moved through the large intestine for elimination.

- The outermost layer is the *serous membrane*. The serous membrane is part of the visceral peritoneum.

Peritoneum

- Most of the abdominal organs of the alimentary canal are covered by the *peritoneum*.

- The peritoneum is a serous membrane composed of simple epithelial cells. The actual name of the peritoneum may change according to the organ it is attached to. The *parietal peritoneum* lines the walls of the abdominal cavity, and the *visceral peritoneum* covers abdominal organs. The space between the two peritoneal layers contains *serous fluid* which facilitates the movement of one organ against another during peristalsis.

- The peritoneum has large folds spaced among the abdominal organs of the alimentary canal and covering organs. These folds or extensions contain numerous blood vessels, lymphatic vessels, and nerves. The folds or extensions from the peritoneum, which hold the small intestine in position, are known as the *mesentery*. The folds extending from the peritoneum, which hold the large intestine in position, make up the *mesocolon*.

- Folds from the peritoneum called the *falciform* hold the liver in place with attachments to the abdominal wall and diaphragm.

- The *greater omentum* extends from the peritoneal folds to cover the front of the intestines and holds the transverse colon and part of small intestine in place. The *lesser omentum* suspends the stomach and duodenum in place.

- The pancreas, duodenum, ascending colon, descending colon, and kidneys lie in the *retroperitoneal space* or behind the peritoneum.

ORGANS OF THE ALIMENTARY CANAL

Mouth and Oral Cavity

- The *mouth* takes in food, which may be in either liquid or solid form, and begins the process of digestion.

- Inside the mouth is the *tongue* which covers the floor. The tongue is a muscular structure which contains the organs of taste and allows movement facilitating the mixing of food with secretions from the salivary glands.

- The upper border or roof of the mouth is called the *palate*. The more anterior portion is known as the *hard palate* because of its bony structure. The posterior portion is the *soft palate* and consists of soft tissue and muscle which provide assistance in swallowing. Hanging from the soft palate is the *uvula*.

- Covering both sides of the throat or pharynx are *tonsils,* which are part of lymphatic tissue that aids in fighting infection.

- Arising from the alveolar processes on the mandible are the *teeth*. The first set of teeth, which appear at about 6 months of age, are the *deciduous teeth* or "baby" teeth. Deciduous teeth are lost between 6 and 12 years of age and are replaced by 32 permanent teeth.

- Teeth are essential in *grinding* and *chewing food* and in mixing secretions from the salivary glands.

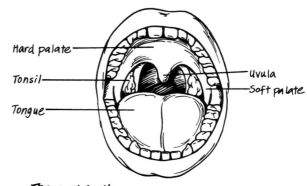

The oral cavity.

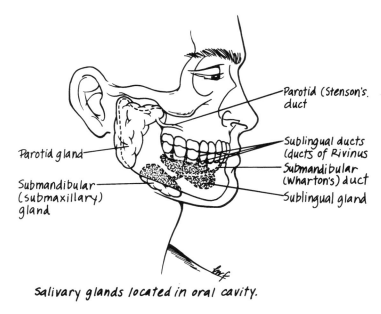

Salivary glands located in oral cavity.

- The *salivary glands* are accessory organs with ducts that open into the mouth. Saliva is the fluid substance produced by these glands, and when mixed with food, it begins the chemical breakdown of food nutrients and digestion.

- There are three pairs of salivary glands, the parotid, sublingual, and submandibular.

- The *parotid glands* are the largest of the salivary glands and are located near the angles of the jaw. The ducts open into the mouth along the upper exterior border of the maxillary molars. In the viral disease *mumps*, the parotid glands become inflamed.

- The smallest of the salivary glands are the *sublingual glands* located on the floor of the mouth and under the tongue, with ducts opening onto the floor of the mouth.

- Located more posteriorly and on the floor of the mouth are the *submandibular glands*, which have ducts (*Wharton's ducts*) that open more anteriorly also on the floor of the mouth.

Pharynx

- The *pharynx* or throat plays a dual role as part of the digestive system and part of the respiratory system. Food passes through it during digestion, and air passes through it during respiration.

- The pharynx is located between the mouth and the esophagus. The upper portion is called the *nasopharynx* and extends from the nasal cavity to the back of the oral cavity, serving as a passageway for air. The middle portion just posterior to the oral cavity is known as the *oropharynx* and serves as a passageway for food and air.

- The lower portion of the pharynx is the *laryngopharynx* and connects the throat to the larynx. This passageway allows food to pass through to the esophagus and air to pass through to the larynx. The larynx has protective mechanisms that prevent food particles from entering the larynx and respiratory system.

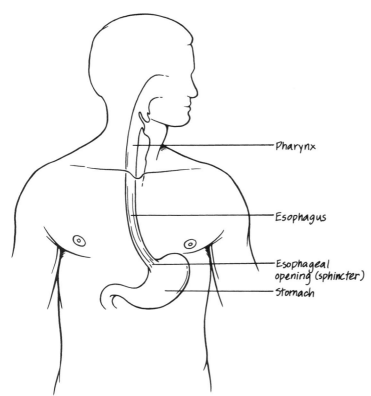

Pharynx

Esophagus

Esophageal opening (sphincter)

Stomach

The esophagus connects superiorly with pharynx and inferiorly with stomach.

Esophagus

- The *esophagus* or *gullet* is a flexible tube connecting the pharynx to the stomach. It is approximately 25 cm (10 in.) in length. The walls of the esophagus are lined with mucosa, and adjacent layers contain muscle tissue which produces peristalsis by which a bolus of food is moved into the stomach.

Stomach

- The *stomach* is a curved, expanded portion of the alimentary canal. The esophagus enters the stomach at the *cardia* or *cardiac region*. The upper portion of the stomach lying superior to the cardia is the *fundus*, and the main expanded portion is the *body* of the stomach. The more distal portion of the stomach is the *pylorus*; it contains the pyloric sphincter, the valve that releases food nutrients or chyme entering the small intestine.

- Along the lateral aspect of the stomach is the *greater curvature,* and the smaller medial curve is the *lesser curvature.*

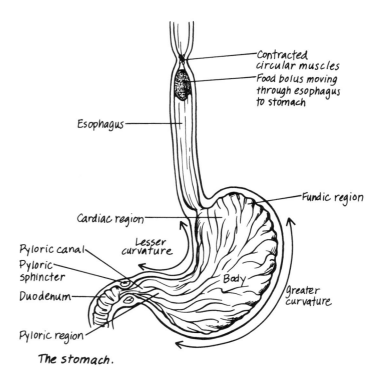

Contracted circular muscles

Food bolus moving through esophagus to stomach

Esophagus

Cardiac region

Pyloric canal

Pyloric sphincter

Duodenum

Pyloric region

Fundic region

Lesser curvature

Body

Greater curvature

The stomach.

- The muscular structure is significant in the "churning" and mixing of food before it enters the small intestine. The inner mucosal layer has large folds called *rugae*. The mucosal lining contains *mucous cells* which secrete mucus, *gastric glands, chief cells,* and other cells that produce gastric secretions to be mixed with food in the stomach.

- The muscular peristaltic movements mix food with enzymes and digestive juices, producing a liquid substance called *chyme*. Chyme is a soft, liquid substance containing food that has been partially digested by digestive juices from the stomach and the salivary glands.

- The gastric juices include mucus which produces an alkaline covering for the walls of the stomach. *Pepsin* is another gastric juice produced in the stomach from pepsinogen as it is stimulated by the presence of other gastric juices and enzymes. *Pepsinogen* is secreted by the gastric glands.

- *Hydrochloric acid* is secreted by parietal cells. The acid environment is necessary for the gastric juices to mix with and break down food substances.

- *Intrinsic factor* is a secretion from the mucosal lining of the stomach and aids in the absorption of vitamin B_{12}.

- The digestive juices produced in the stomach supply an acid environment, and the alkaline mucus provides a covering for the walls of the stomach so that the digestive process does not destroy or break down these walls.

- The regulation of gastric secretions is under the control of the parasympathetic nervous system.

Small Intestine

- The *small intestine* is the flexible tube that receives chyme from the pyloric region of the stomach. The small intestine is just over 6 m (21 ft) in length and provides a vast surface for the absorption of digested food nutrients.

- The small intestine is divided into three parts called the duodenum, jejunum, and ileum.

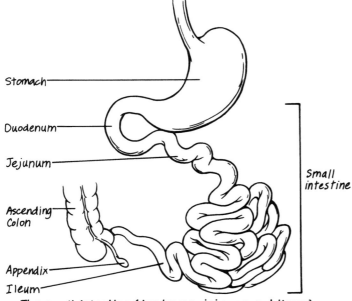

Stomach

Duodenum

Jejunum

Ascending Colon

Appendix

Ileum

Small intestine

The small intestine (duodenum, jejunum and ileum).

- The liver, pancreas, and gallbladder are *accessory organs* with ducts opening into the proximal portion of the small intestine.

- The *duodenum* is the most proximal portion of the small intestine. It is a C-shaped structure about 25 cm (10 in.) in length. It connects proximally with the pylorus and distally with the jejunum.

- The *jejunum* lies between the duodenum and ileum and has a length of about 2.5 m.

- The distal end of the small intestine is the *ileum* and is about 3.5 m long. It enters the large intestine at the *ileocecal valve*, a muscle sphincter that controls the movement of material from the small intestine to the large intestine.

- The mucosal lining of the small intestine is slightly different from that of the stomach because absorption is the primary activity in this part of the alimentary canal. Long, tiny villi project outward, providing a greater surface for absorption.

- The *intestinal villi* contain glands that secrete digestive enzymes needed for the further breakdown of food materials. The small intestine functions to absorb carbohydrates, fats, and proteins.

- Materials are moved through the small intestine by peristalsis.

Accessory Organs Associated with the Small Intestine

- The *accessory organs* associated with the small intestine are the liver, gallbladder, and pancreas.

- The *liver* is a large organ and fills much of the right hypochrondiac region of the abdominal cavity. It is a wedge-shaped organ extending across the midline into the epigastrium. On the lateral aspect the liver dips to near the level of the right kidney.

- The liver is divided into two major lobes. The *right* lobe is the large lobe, and the *left* lobe is the smaller lobe.

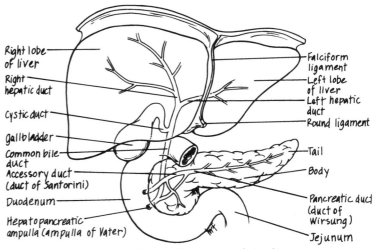

Pancreas in relation to liver, gallbladder and duodenum.

- The functions of the liver include *carbohydrate, fat, and protein metabolism; production and storage of glycogen; and storage of vitamins A, D, and B$_{12}$ and iron*. The liver forms and secretes bile, which is a waste product of red blood cell destruction. Although bile is a waste product, it is used in the digestion of fats. Excretion of bile formed in the liver takes place through the bile ducts and the gallbladder. The duct that exits the liver is the *common hepatic duct*.

- The *gallbladder* is a storage reservoir for bile. It is a pear-shaped organ resting under the liver but hanging freely. The gallbladder holds bile, allowing it to be stored in a more concentrated form. Following contractions stimulated by the presence of fat, the gallbladder releases bile into the *cystic duct*.

- The common hepatic duct and the cystic duct join to form the *common bile duct*.

- The pancreas is a long gland (12 to 13 cm or about 5 in.) which lies mostly horizontally in the posterior abdominal cavity. The head of the pancreas rests in the C-loop of the duodenum.

- The pancreas functions as both an *endocrine gland*, by secreting the hormone insulin, and as a *digestive accessory organ (exocrine gland)*, by secreting pancreatic juices needed for digestion. Pancreatic juices provide an alkaline environment which interrupts the activity of pepsin. The alkaline environment is needed for the small intestine to absorb and further break down food substances.

- Pancreatic juices empty into the pancreatic duct or the *duct of Wirsung*.

- The duct of Wirsung and the common bile duct form the *hepatopancreatic ampulla* or the *ampulla of Vater*. The ampulla of Vater empties into the duodenum through the *sphincter of Oddi*.

Large Intestine

- The distal end of the alimentary canal is the *large intestine*. It is approximately 1.5 m (5 ft) in length and functions in digestion to complete *absorption* (especially the absorption of water to maintain a water balance in the body) and in forming feces. The large intestine also functions in the *elimination* of fecal waste material.

- The mucosal lining of the large intestine differs from that of the small intestine. No villi are present, and the muscular layer is more prominent. The muscular layer is capable of producing the strong peristaltic waves needed to push feces through the intestine for elimination.

- The most proximal portion of the large intestine is the slightly expanded *cecum* located just inferior to the opening for the *ileocecal valve*. Extending from the medial surface of the cecum is the *vermiform appendix*.

- Above the cecum is the *ascending colon,* which bends anteriorly at the *hepatic flexure* to become the *transverse colon*. The transverse colon dips as it crosses the abdominal cavity to the *splenic flexure* where it bends posteriorly to become the *descending colon*. At the end of the descending colon is the S-shaped *sigmoid colon.*

- Distal to the sigmoid colon and situated more vertically and posteriorly is the *rectum*. The rectum leads to the lower *anal canal* and the exterior opening called the *anus*. The process of emptying the rectum is called *defecation.*

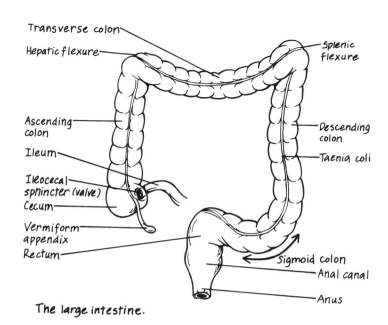

The large intestine.

PATHOPHYSIOLOGIC TERMINOLOGY ASSOCIATED WITH THE DIGESTIVE SYSTEM

Achalasia failure of the esophageal sphincter muscle to relax completely and permit food to move into the stomach

Ankyloglossia condition in which a person is tongue-tied

Anorexia loss of appetite

Appendicitis an inflammation of the appendix

Ascites an accumulation of fluid in the abdominal cavity

Bulimia gorging of food following by self-induced vomiting

Cholecystitis an inflammation of the gallbladder

Cholelithiasis the presence of stones or calculi in the gallbladder

Cirrhosis destructive liver disease

Colitis an inflammation of the colon

Crohn's disease a chronic inflammatory disease of the lower gastrointestinal tract

Diarrhea frequent elimination of feces; loss of water may result, causing dehydration

Diverticulitis an inflammation of diverticula or pouches found in the intestines

Diverticulosis a condition characterized by pouches or small sacs which arise from the walls of the intestine

Dyspepsia indigestion
Enteritis an inflammation of the small intestine
Fistula abnormal opening between two organs
Gastritis an inflammation of the stomach lining
Gastroenteritis an inflammation of the intestines and the stomach
Hepatitis an inflammation of the liver; may be due to toxins or a virus; characterized by jaundice and enlargement of the liver
Hepatomegaly enlargement of the liver
Hiatal hernia condition in which a portion of the stomach protrudes through the esophageal opening in the diaphragm
Ileitis an inflammation of the ileum
Pancreatitis an inflammation of the pancreas
Peptic ulcer destruction of the mucous membrane in either the stomach or the duodenum; if untreated it will result in a lesion or ulcer.

Chapter 9 Practice Questions

1. Which of the following is an accessory organ of the alimentary canal?
   a. spleen
   b. adrenal gland
   c. thymus gland
   d. pancreas

2. Contractions of muscles, both longitudinal and circular, that push food through the alimentary canal are called
   a. peritoneum movements.
   b. peristalsis.
   c. mesenteric movements.
   d. mastication

3. The abdominal cavity is lined with a serous membrane called the
   a. peritoneum.
   b. omentum.
   c. mesenteric.
   d. viseral mesenteric.

4. The extension of the peritoneum that stretches over the front of the intestines is the
   a. mesocolon.
   b. retroperitoneum.
   c. greater omentum.
   d. lesser omentum.

5. Glands located in the oral cavity that secrete substances that initiate the breakdown of food particles are called
   a. Wharton's ducts.
   b. mucosal glands.
   c. salivary glands.
   d. deciduous glands.

6. The flap on the superior portion of the larynx that prevents food from entering the respiratory system is the
   a. gullet.
   b. epiglottis.
   c. laryngopharynx.
   d. glottis.

7. The liquid substance produced by the mixing of food in the stomach is called
   a. chyme.
   b. pepsin.
   c. pepsinogen.
   d. intrinsic factor.

8. The smallest section of the small intestine is the
   a. duodenum.
   b. jejunum.
   c. ileum.
   d. ileocecum.

9. The portion of the large intestine located just beneath the liver is the
   a. ileocecal region.
   b. hepatic flexure.
   c. splenic flexure.
   d. sigmoid colon.

10. Which of the following ducts releases bile and pancreatic juices into the duodenum?
   a. common bile duct
   b. common hepatic duct
   c. cystic duct
   d. ampulla of Vater

The Cardiovascular System

- The organs and tissue that make up the *cardiovascular system* are the *heart, blood vessels,* and *blood.*

BLOOD

- *Blood* is a type of connective tissue with *cell*s suspended in a liquid material called *plasma.* The adult body contains about 5 L of blood.

- Whole blood is more viscous than water. Blood plasma serves as a suspension for red blood cells, white blood cells, and platelets.

Red Blood Cells

- *Red blood cells,* also called *erythrocytes,* are small, round cells with a concave surface on each side. The biconcave surface provides a thin center section. *Hemoglobin* is part of red blood cells and is mainly located in the center section, serving as the agent for transporting oxygen to cells throughout the body. When oxygen is present in the hemoglobin, the blood appears bright red.

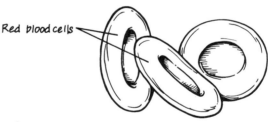

Red blood cells.

- Hemoglobin also contains iron and protein, which are recycled in the formation of new red blood cells.

- *Mature red blood cells* do not have a nucleus. A nucleus is present in a young, developing red blood cell but disappears as the cell matures. A normal red blood cell lives for approximately 120 days.

- A normal adult has approximately 4 to 6 million red blood cells per cubic millimeter. Males have a slightly higher red blood cell count. Since red blood cells provide oxygen to cells, if the number of cells drops, the oxygen-carrying capacity also drops.

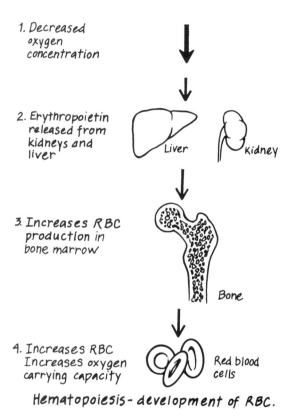

1. Decreased oxygen concentration

2. Erythropoietin released from kidneys and liver

   Liver   Kidney

3. Increases RBC production in bone marrow

   Bone

4. Increases RBC Increases oxygen carrying capacity   Red blood cells

Hematopoiesis - development of RBC.

- Red blood cells must be flexible in order to turn and move through tiny blood vessels and capillaries.

- As red blood cells become damaged, they are destroyed in the liver and spleen by macrophages and new red blood cells are produced. Red blood cells are formed in the red bone marrow of the skeleton.

- As old or damaged red blood cells are destroyed, the iron and protein contained in the cells are recycled for use in the production of new red blood cells. Excess iron and protein can be stored in the liver as *biliverdin*. Biliverdin is later changed into an orange pigment called *bilirubin*. Both biliverdin and bilirubin are excreted in bile.

- Red blood cell formation, known as *hematopoiesis*, takes place in the vascular tissue of the red bone marrow. The process of cell formation is stimulated by a negative feedback system. As the hemoglobin or red blood cell count drops, *erythropoietin*, a hormone that initiates formation of more red blood cells, is released from the kidney.

- Red blood cell production is facilitated by the presence of vitamin B12, folic acid, and iron. A deficiency in any of these nutrients affects the formation of new red blood cells.

- *Anemia* is a deficiency in the number of red blood cells or in hemoglobin. Common types of anemia are hypochromic anemia, aplastic anemia, hemolytic anemia, pernicious anemia, and hemorrhagic anemia.

- *Hypochromic anemia* is caused by an insufficiency of iron.

- *Aplastic anemia* is related to the inability of the red bone marrow to develop new cells.

- *Hemolytic anemia* results when red blood cell membranes begin to rupture.

- *Pernicious anemia* is caused by insufficient production of red blood cells, which in turn prevents the absorption of B_{12} in the stomach.

- *Hemorrhagic anemia* is caused by excessive loss of red blood cells as a result of blood loss.

Red Blood Cells and Blood Type

- The presence of certain substances in a person's blood identifies the blood type. There are two substances, called *agglutinogen A* and *agglutinogen B,* that may be present in a person's red blood cells. In the blood plasma the associated antibodies are called *agglutinins.*

- The presence of agglutinogen A in a red blood cell is associated with *blood type A.* Associated with agglutinogen A is the presence of the agglutinin *anti-B* in the plasma.

- The presence of agglutinogen B is associated with blood *type B.* Associated with blood type B is the agglutinin *anti-A* in the plasma.

- Both agglutinogens A and B can be present, producing the blood *type AB.* For blood type AB, there are no agglutinins in the plasma.

- When no agglutinogens are present in the red blood cells, the blood type is *type O.* For blood type O, the associated agglutinins in the plasma are both anti-A and anti-B.

- For a blood transfusion, the blood type must be matched as closely as possible to prevent reactions caused by the antibodies in the plasma.

- In the transfusion of blood, individuals with type O blood, which has no agglutinogens, are called *universal donors.*

- Individuals with type AB blood, which has no agglutinins in the plasma, are known as *universal recipients.*

- The *Rh factor* is another component of blood type. If this factor is present, the blood type is *Rh-positive*, and if it is not present, the blood type is *Rh-negative. Erythroblastosis fetalis* may occur when a mother is Rh-negative and the fetus she is carrying is Rh-positive.

White Blood Cells

- *White blood cells* or *leukocytes* are divided into two types called *granulocytes* and *agranulocytes.* Their major function is to develop and support the body's *immune system* and *fight infection.*

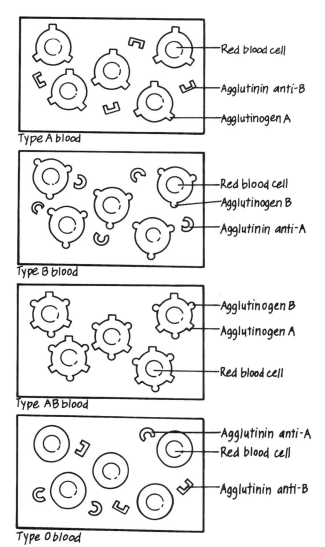

Blood types A, B, AB and O with agglutinogens and agglutinins

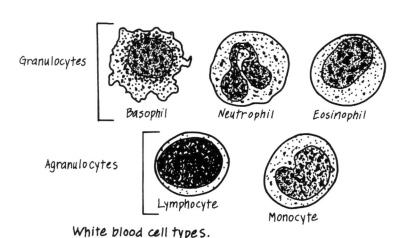

White blood cell types.

- The total number of white blood cells in an adult human is about 5000 to 10,000 per cubic milliliter. The white blood cell count may vary if an infection is present somewhere in the body. In general, the number of white blood cells rises in the presence of an infection, increasing the number of cells available to attack invading microorganisms.

- An insufficient number of white blood cells (less than 5000 per cubic milliliter) is called *leukopenia*, and an excess number of white blood cells is called *eukocytosis*.

Granulocytes

- *Granulocytes* are so called because of the appearance of granules in the cytoplasm. The types of granulocytes include neutrophils, eosinophils, and basophils.

- The function of *neutrophils* is phagocytosis. They make up over 50 percent of the total number of white blood cells.

- *Eosinophils* make up about 3 percent of the total white blood cell count and function in controlling inflammation and allergic reactions.

- *Basophils* make up about 1 percent of the total white blood cell count and function in the release of heparin and histamine.

Agranulocytes

- Agranulocytes do not have granular cytoplasm, and the two types are monocytes and lymphocytes. *Monocytes* make up about 7 to 9 percent of the total white blood cell count, and their main function is to phagocytize large particles.

- *Lymphocytes* compose about 25 percent of the total white blood cell count and serve as a major source of immunity. Some lymphocytes are capable of forming antibodies and help in the prevention of infection and disease.

PLATELETS

- *Blood platelets* or *thrombocytes* originate in the red bone marrow and appear as immature cells. They have no nucleus and are much smaller than red blood cells. Under normal conditions there are 130,000 to 360,000 platelets per cubic millimeter. The primary function of blood platelets is to facilitate the *clotting of blood* and stopping the loss of blood, thus maintaining *hemostasis.*

BLOOD PLASMA

- *Plasma* is about 90 percent water and is the liquid part of blood. Components of the plasma liquid include organic and inorganic materials.

- Types of *protein* found in plasma are albumin, globulin, and fibrinogen. *Albumin* aids in maintaining cellular osmotic pressure.

- *Globulins* aid in the transportation of lipids and fat-soluble vitamins. *Gamma globulins* are the antibodies of immunity in the body.

- *Fibrinogen* plays a key role along with platelets in the formation of blood clots **to** prevent blood loss.

- Other nutrients found in plasma are amino acids, sugars, and lipids being transported to tissues and cells. In addition, plasma contains nitrogen and electrolytes.

THE CIRCULATORY SYSTEM: HEART AND BLOOD VESSELS

- The *heart* and *blood vessels* move blood to all parts of the body. The heart serves as the pump that forces the blood through the arteries, capillaries, and veins. *Arteries* are larger muscular vessels which carry blood away from the heart. Arteries carry oxygenated blood, except for the pulmonary arteries, and veins carry deoxygenated blood, except for the pulmonary veins. *Arterioles* and *capillaries* are small vessels that carry blood and nutrients to cells.

- *Venules* are small veins that drain blood from cells and tissues, emptying into larger *veins* which transport blood back to the heart.

- The walls of capillaries are semipermeable to facilitate the exchange of blood gases and nutrients to support cellular metabolism.

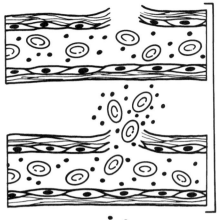

As blood escapes through break in blood vessel, red blood cells and platelets will escape.

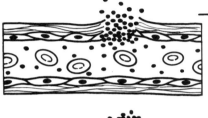

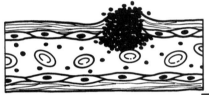

Platelets begin to stick to each other and form a plug (clot) closing off the break and preventing loss of blood.

Platelets' role in forming a blood clot to stop loss of blood.

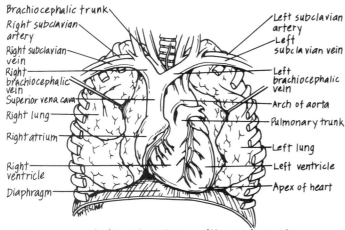

Anterior aspect of heart and lungs with great vessels.

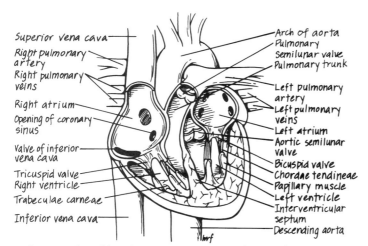

Cross section of heart showing right and left ventricles, right and left atria, valves and major vessels.

Heart

- The *heart* is a cone-shaped structure about the size of a large fist. Inside the heart are four hollow chambers. The heart is located just behind the sternum and is slightly tilted, resting on the diaphragm.

- The *apex* of the heart is the pointed end that rests on the diaphragm, and the *base* is the upper portion where major blood vessels exit the heart.

- The heart is covered by a double-layered fibrous membrane called the *pericardium*. The outer layer is the *fibrous pericardium,* and the inner layer is the *visceral pericardium* (epicardium). The two layers are separated by the *pericardial cavity.*

- The *epicardium* serves as the outer layer of the heart structure.

- The middle layer of heart tissue is the *myocardium* and contains specialized heart muscle tissue which produces the sequence of contractions that pump blood through the heart. The myocardium contains the blood supply and nerves for the heart. The inner layer of tissue is the endocardium.

- The *endocardium* is composed of connective tissue which includes elastic fibers. Specialized fibers in the endocardium called *Purkinje fibers* play an important role in contraction of the heart muscle.

- Within the heart are *four chambers*. The two upper chambers are the *right atrium* and *left atrium*, and the lower and larger chambers are the *right ventricle* and *left ventricle.*

- The right atrium and the right ventricle are separated from the left side of the heart by a *septum*. Each atrium is connected to the ventricle below it by a specialized heart valve.

- The valve between the right atrium and the right ventricle is the *tricuspid* valve. It has three cusps that allow blood to move from the right atrium to the right ventricle but not in the opposite direction. When the valve is functioning properly, blood does not leak back into the atrium.

- The valve between the left atrium and the left ventricle is the *bicuspid* or *mitral valve* and has only two cusps. This valve allows blood to move only from the atrium to the ventricle and not in the opposite direction.

- The right ventricle has a thinner muscular wall. Blood leaving the right ventricle is sent to the lungs for oxygen and carbon dioxide exchange. The opening from the right ventricle through which blood leaves the heart is the *pulmonary semilunar* valve, which has three cusps. The blood leaves the right ventricle and enters the *pulmonary trunk* which branches into the pulmonary arteries. The blood in the pulmonary arteries is unoxygenated blood.

- The right atrium has openings on the posterior wall through which the *superior* and *inferior venae cavae* and *coronary sinuses* empty blood into the heart.

- As the blood leaves the left ventricle, it passes through the *aortic semilunar valve* into the *aorta.*

- The left atrium has openings through which *pulmonary veins* empty oxygenated blood from the lungs into the heart.

Blood Circulation through the Heart and Lungs

- Blood enters the heart as unoxygenated blood through the venae cavae and coronary sinus. The blood circulates through the heart taking the following path:

  Right atrium
    through the tricuspid valve
    Right ventricle
    through the pulmonary semilunar valve
  Pulmonary trunk
  Pulmonary artery
    Arterioles to capillaries for oxygen and carbon
      dioxide exchange
    Venules to pulmonary veins
    Left atrium
    through the bicuspid or mitral valve
    Left ventricle
    through the semilunar valve
  Aorta

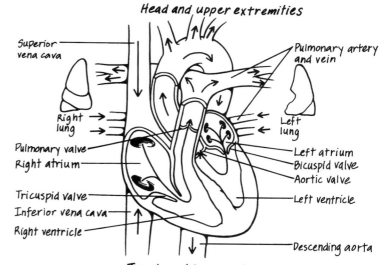

Circulation of blood through heart and lungs.

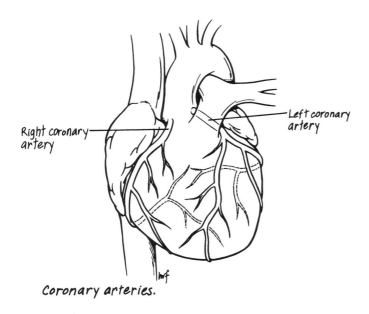

Right coronary artery

Left coronary artery

Coronary arteries.

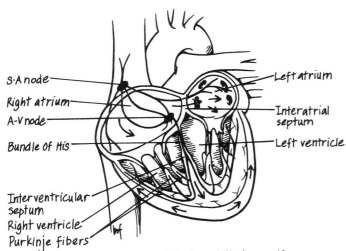

S-A node

Right atrium

A-V node

Bundle of His

Interventricular septum

Right ventricle

Purkinje fibers

Left atrium

Interatrial septum

Left ventricle

The conduction system of the heart that results in cardiac contraction.

Coronary Circulation

- Blood is supplied to the heart by the *right* and *left coronary arteries*. The first branches from the aorta are the coronary arteries. The coronary arteries and capillaries supply oxygen and nutrients to the myocardium and other heart tissue.

- When the coronary arteries or capillaries become constricted or clogged as a result of arteriosclerotic disease, the oxygenated blood supply is decreased, producing *ischemia*. Pain associated with ischemia is known as *angina pectoris* and is felt in the chest area. Extreme ischemic conditions may produce a *myocardial infarct* (a heart attack).

The Heart Muscle and Contractions

- Blood is moved through the heart by a *sequence of contractions* which force it from one chamber to another.

- The *cardiac cycle* first involves contraction of the atrial walls while the ventricular walls relax. This part of the cycle creates greater pressure in the atrium, pushing blood into the ventricles. During the next part of the cycle the ventricular walls contract and the atrial walls relax. Since special valves prevent the blood from returning to the atria, it is pushed through the valve openings in each of the ventricles. When the atrial walls relax, blood from the venae cavae and coronary sinuses empties into the right atrium and blood from the lungs fills the left atrium.

- The contractions result from actions of specialized muscle tissue. The conducting cycle begins at the *sinoatrial (S-A) node* which is called the heart's *pacemaker*. These specialized muscles contract without stimulation.

- After beginning at the S-A node the impulse then moves to activate the *atrioventricular (A-V) node*. First, the S-A node initiates atrial contraction, and then the A-V node initiates ventricular contraction. To achieve ventricular contraction the impulse must move through the *A-V bundle,* also called the *bundle of His,* and the *Purkinje fibers* which are spread throughout the inner walls of the ventricles.

- An *electrocardiogram* (ECG) is a recording of the heart's conducting system.

- The waveform has a specific P-QRS-T pattern. The *P wave* represents depolarization of the atrium, the *QRS wave* represents depolarization of the ventricles and repolarization of the atria, and the *T* wave represents repolarization of the ventricles. This wave pattern occurs about 60 to 80 times a minute with normal activity.

- *Tachycardia* is a heartbeat of more than 100 beats per minute. *Bradycardia* is a heartbeat of less than 60 beats per minute. *Heart flutter* refers to erratic, rapid, incomplete contractions of the heart.

Blood Vessels

- The *blood vessels* form a closed system for blood circulation. *Arteries* are the strong elastic vessels that can withstand the pressure of the heart pushing oxygenated blood through the vascular system.

- Arteries branch into *arterioles* which continue branching into capillaries.

- *Capillaries* are the smallest blood vessels and are semipermeable in order to facilitate the movement of substances across the membranes of the vessels. Movement is by osmosis, diffusion, or filtration.

- Capillaries return blood through small *venules* which in turn empty into larger *veins*. Veins move deoxygenated blood from the cells to the heart. They are generally larger vessels with valves located throughout the system. In the venous system valves serve as mechanisms to keep blood moving in the proper direction. The pressure from the heart is less in the veins, and therefore it is more difficult for blood to move back toward the heart.

Blood Pressure

- As the heart pumps, pressure is exerted on the walls of the heart and of the blood vessels.

- In the heart *atrial systole* is the maximum pressure applied to the walls of the atrium as it contracts. *Atrial diastole* is the existing pressure when the walls of the atrium relax.

- Pressure in the ventricles during contractions is referred to as *ventricular systole,* and during relaxation as *ventricular diastole.*

- *Arterial blood pressure* is the maximum pressure measured during ventricular contraction and is known as *systolic pressure.* When the ventricle relaxes, the existing pressure in the arteries is the *diastolic pressure.* For example, 120/70 means the systolic pressure is 120 and the diastolic pressure is 70.

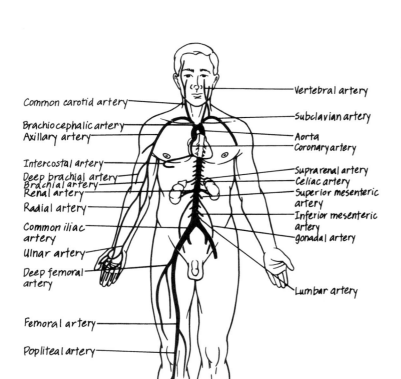

Common carotid artery

Brachiocephalic artery
Axillary artery

Intercostal artery
Deep brachial artery
Brachial artery
Renal artery

Radial artery

Common iliac artery

Ulnar artery

Deep femoral artery

Femoral artery

Popliteal artery

Posterior tibial artery
Anterior tibial artery
Peroneal artery

Dorsal pedis artery

Vertebral artery
Subclavian artery
Aorta
Coronary artery
Suprarenal artery
Celiac artery
Superior mesenteric artery
Inferior mesenteric artery
gonadal artery

Lumbar artery

The aorta and major arterial branches.

MAJOR BLOOD VESSELS IMPORTANT IN RADIOGRAPHIC PROCEDURES

- The major arteries branching from the aorta, beginning with the ascending aorta, are the *coronary arteries, brachiocephalic artery, left common carotid artery,* and *left subclavian branch from the aortic arch.* The aorta descends through the thorax and into the abdominal cavity. In the abdominal cavity are the *celiac artery* branching just inferiorly to the diaphragm, the *renal arteries,* and the *superior* and *inferior mesenteric arteries.*

- As the aorta enters the lower abdominal cavity and pelvis it branches into the right and left *common iliac arteries.*

- The major blood vessels that supply blood to the brain are the *right* and *left common carotid* and *vertebral arteries.* The right common carotid artery branches from the brachiocephalic artery, and the left common carotid artery branches directly from the aortic arch.

- The blood supply to the upper extremities is provided by the *subclavian arteries,* which branch into the *axillary, brachial, radial,* and *ulnar arteries.*

- The blood supply to the lower extremities is supplied by the *common iliac arteries,* which branch into the *femoral, popliteal,* and *tibial arteries.*

- The *celiac artery* branches into the *hepatic artery* to supply the liver, into the *gastric artery* to supply the upper gastrointestinal tract, and into the *splenic artery* to supply the spleen.

- The *superior* and *inferior mesenteric arteries* provide the large and small intestines with blood, and the *renal arteries* supply blood to the kidneys.

- Venous blood is drained from the head via the *jugular veins*. Veins with names corresponding to those of the arteries empty blood from all parts of the body.

- The *hepatic portal venous system* is unique and drains blood from the abdominal gastrointestinal tract through the liver. The gastric veins from the stomach and superior and inferior mesenteric veins empty blood from the large and small intestines. The splenic vein empties blood from the spleen. The *gastric, mesenteric,* and *splenic veins empty into the hepatic portal vein* which circulates the blood to the liver. From the liver blood is emptied into the venae cavae by the *hepatic vein*.

- The lower extremities are drained by the *femoral, saphenous, popliteal,* and *tibial* veins.

PATHOPHYSIOLOGIC TERMINOLOGY ASSOCIATED WITH THE BLOOD AND THE CIRCULATORY SYSTEM

Blood

Anemia a deficiency of hemoglobin or red blood cells; can have a variety of origins

Infectious mononucleosis a contagious disease involving lymphatic tissue and blood; results in an increase in white blood cells and especially in the number of lymphocytes

Leukemia a malignant disease of blood tissue; may be chronic or acute; characterized by the uncontrolled production of leukocytes; acute leukemia may cause internal hemorrhaging

Monocytopenia a decreased monocyte count

Multiple myeloma a malignancy involving plasma cells in bone marrow.

Neutropenia a decreased neutrophil count

Polycythemia an increased blood hematocrit (percentage of blood consisting of red blood cells) causing increased blood viscosity

Polycythemia vera an excess of red blood cells present because of an increase in total blood volume

Septicemia systemic blood poisoning usually of bacterial origin

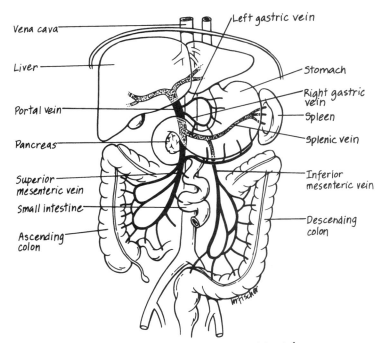

The hepatic portal system drains venous blood from gastrointestinal tract.

Sickle cell anemia an inherited disorder causing red blood cells to be sickle-shaped, which prevents them from moving through small blood vessels; as the red blood cells change in shape, they can be easily ruptured as they move through the circulatory system.

Circulatory System

Aneurysm a blood-filled sac formed by stretching of the wall of a blood vessel

Aortic insufficiency a condition in which blood from the aorta leaks backward into the left ventricle because of a faulty aortic semilunar valve

Aortic stenosis a narrowing of the aorta

Arrhythmia a disruption of the normal rhythm of the heartbeat

Atherosclerosis a condition in which the walls of blood vessels are embedded with plaques containing fat and cholesterol

Cardiomegaly enlargement of the heart

Congestive heart failure a condition in which the heart is unable to maintain blood flow over a prolonged period of time, causing poor circulation and edema

Cyanosis a bluish color of the skin caused by a lack of hemoglobin

Embolism the blocking of a blood vessel by a clot or possibly by an air bubble

Endocarditis an inflammation of the inner lining of the heart

Heart block a partial or complete disruption of the cardiac conducting system

Hemangioma a benign tumor of a cluster of blood vessels

Hematoma blood that has accumulated in tissue and formed a clot

Hemoptysis spitting up blood

Hypertension high blood pressure

Hypotension low blood pressure

Mitral stenosis narrowing of the mitral valve

Mitral valve prolapse a disorder associated with displacement of the mitral valve during contraction of the heart, causing the valve cusps to be stretched

Myocarditis an inflammation of the heart muscle

Occlusion a closing off or obstruction of a blood vessel

Pericarditis an inflammation of the pericardium around the heart

Phlebitis an inflammation of the veins

Thrombophlebitis an inflammation of a vein with clot formation

Thrombosis a blood clot

Varicose chronic swelling of veins

Chapter 10 Practice Questions

1. The type of blood cell that serves as the transport mechanism for hemoglobin is a (an)

   a. erythrocyte.
   b. leukocyte.
   c. eosinophil.
   d. thrombocyte.

2. A deficiency in the number of red blood cells or hemoglobin is referred to as

   a. hemostasis.
   b. erythrocytosis.
   c. anemia.
   d. erythroblastosis.

3. A person with which of the following blood types is known as a universal donor?

   a. type A
   b. type B
   c. type AB
   d. type O

4. Granulocytes that function as phagocytes are called

   a. neutrophils.
   b. basophils.
   c. eosinophils.
   d. erythrocytes.

5. What type of blood cell maintains hemostasis by facilitating the clotting of blood?

   a. leukocytes
   b. erythrocytes
   c. platelets
   d. globulins

6. Vessels that transport blood away from the heart are called

   a. arteries.
   b. veins.
   c. lymphatics.
   d. venules.

7. The opening between the left atrium and left ventricle is the

   a. bicuspid valve.
   b. tricuspid valve.
   c. pulmonary semilunar valve.
   d. aortic semilunar valve.

8. The chamber of the heart with the thickest muscular layer is the
   a. left atrium.
   b. right atrium.
   c. left ventricle.
   d. right ventricle.

9. Blood empties into the heart from the
   a. descending aorta.
   b. vena cava.
   c. carotid veins.
   d. hepatic portal system.

10. The maximum pressure exerted on the walls of the arteries during ventricular contraction is the _____ pressure.
    a. arterial blood
    b. ventricular systolic
    c. systolic
    d. diastolic

The Lymphatic System

- The *lymphatic system* is closely associated with the cardiovascular system and functions to *transport fluid* from cells to the circulatory system. In addition to being involved in transportation, the lymphatic system plays an important role in *immunity* and helps *fight infection*.

- Lymphatic vessels are similar in structure to blood vessels but do not form a closed system. These vessels originate in the interstitial spaces with *closed-end lymphatic capillaries*. The small lymphatic capillaries join other lymph capillaries to form larger vessels which lead to *lymphatic ducts*.

- There are two major lymphatic ducts called the *thoracic* or *left lymphatic duct* and the *right lymphatic duct*. Both of these ducts collect lymph fluid from tissues throughout the body and empty it into the blood via veins in the thoracic cavity.

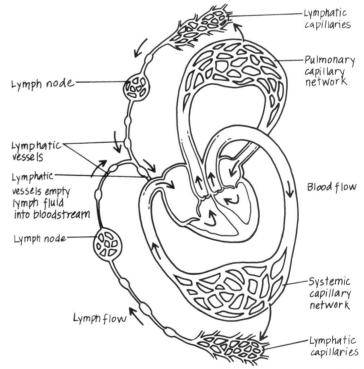

Lymphatic network parallels blood vessel network emptying tissue fluid (lymph) into blood stream.

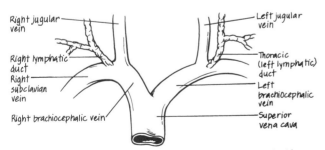

Right and left (thoracic) lymphatic ducts empty lymph fluid into venous blood flow.

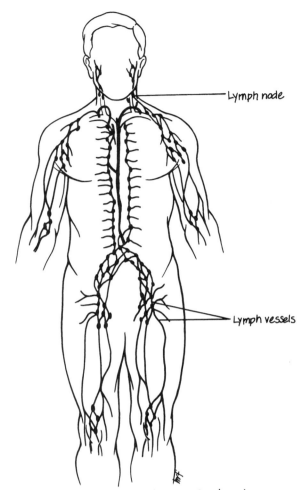

Lymph node and lymphatic vessel network.

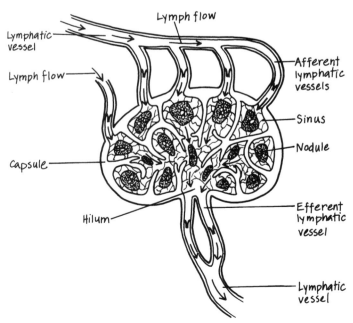

Lymph node structure indicating lymph node.

- Lymphatic ducts empty lymph fluid into the venous system where it mixes and circulates with blood. Located throughout the lymphatic system are clusters of *lymph nodes* composed of lymphatic tissue.

- Lymph fluid contains proteins which are to be returned to the bloodstream.

- The lymph system has no source of pressure to force lymph fluid through the lymphatic vessels; therefore, the movement of skeletal muscles must provide sufficient force to move this fluid.

Lymph Nodes

- Lymph nodes located along the lymphatic pathways contain a large number of lymphocytes. Lymph fluid passes through the nodes where it is filtered and microorganisms are attacked and destroyed by the lymphocytes.

- Lymph nodes are bean-shaped structures with sinuses and nodules and resemble sponges. The structure of the nodes facilitates the filtering process. Lymph enters a node from the lymphatic duct through the afferent lymph vessels and exits in the area of the hilum via efferent lymphatic vessels.

- The lymphatic system may become a primary route for cancer cells to spread to other parts of the body. These cells may break away from the primary tumor and, if picked up by the lymphatic system, spread first to the lymph nodes and eventually to another organ.

- Other lymphatic organs are the *thymus gland*, *spleen*, and *tonsils*.

Thymus Gland

- The *thymus gland* is located in the thoracic cavity in front of the aorta and behind the sternum. The thymus contains lymphocytes which develop into *T lymphocytes* or *T cells* and then move into the circulatory system to become about 75 percent of all circulating lymphocytes. T lymphocytes attack antigens, thus providing immunity.

- Lymphocytes released by the bone marrow that do not reach the thymus gland become *B lymphocytes* or *B cells*, making up the remaining 25 percent of circulating lymphocytes. B cells are found in the lymph nodes and the spleen and function in the production of antibodies which act against antigens.

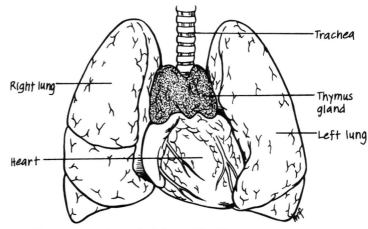

Thymus gland located in mediastinum.

The Spleen

- The *spleen* is located in the left upper quadrant behind the stomach. The tissue in the spleen is similar to lymphatic tissue, with sinuses and nodules. The sinuses in the spleen, however, are filled with blood instead of lymph and function as *blood reservoirs*.

- The spleen contains a significant number of *phagocytes* which are able to eat and destroy bacteria and other invading microorganisms. Microphages in the spleen also destroy damaged red blood cells.

Tonsils

- The *tonsils* are made up of lymphatic tissue surrounded by mucous membrane and are located in the posterior area of the oral cavity where it joins the pharynx. Their major function is to act on microorganisms taken in by the mouth or through the nasal cavity.

Immunity

- When the body is exposed to antigens, antibodies may be produced for several weeks. Some of the T cells and B cells act as memory cells and remain dormant, supporting the development of immunity.

- Immunity is also acquired by the injection of a dead or weakened pathogen into the body, such as a vaccine. Antibodies are formed, producing an acquired active immunity.

- *Acquired immune deficiency syndrome* (AIDS) is caused by a virus that infects the macrophages and T-helper cells. *T-helper cells* are activators of B cells, which produce antibodies and signal macrophages to act on antigens. The AIDS virus can kill T-helper cells, leaving the body with significantly reduced acquired immunity.

PATHOPHYSIOLOGIC TERMINOLOGY ASSOCIATED WITH THE LYMPHATIC SYSTEM

Adenitis an inflammation of the lymph nodes

Hodgkin's lymphoma a neoplastic disease of lymphatic tissue involving the lymph nodes and spleen; usually begins in the neck and spreads throughout the body

Lymphangitis an inflammation of the lymphatic vessels

Lymphedema an accumulation of lymph fluid in subcutaneous tissue causing swelling

Splenomegaly an enlargement of the spleen

Chapter 11 Practice Questions

1. **Which of the following is the primary function of the lymphatic system?**

   a. building immunity to disease
   b. developing lymph nodes
   c. movement of lymph fluid
   d. destruction of old blood cells

2. **Lymphocytes that reside in the thymus gland become _____ and function in the attack on antigens to provide immunity.**

   a. mast cells
   b. macrophages
   c. T lymphocytes
   d. B lymphocytes

3. **Neoplastic disease of the lymphatic tissue involving the lymph nodes and spreading throughout the body is called**

   a. lymphedema.
   b. lymphangitis.
   c. adenitis.
   d. Hodgkin's lymphoma.

4. **The condition in which a virus infects macrophages and T lymphocytes, eventually destroying the immune system, is called**

    a. autoimmune disease.
    b. lymphomegaly.
    c. lymphangioma.
    d. acquired immune deficiency syndrome.

5. **Which of the following organs of the lymphatic system help destroy damaged red blood cells?**

    a. thymus
    b. spleen
    c. lymph nodes
    d. lymphatic ducts

The Respiratory System

THE RESPIRATORY SYSTEM

- The organs of the *respiratory system* are designed to *take in oxygen* and *eliminate carbon dioxide*. Oxygen is necessary for cellular metabolism, and carbon dioxide is a metabolic waste product to be eliminated. The exchange of oxygen and carbon dioxide is called *respiration*. The actual exchange of these gases at the cellular level is referred to as *cellular respiration*.

- The respiratory system also functions in *filtering* and *cleansing air* as it enters the system and in *warming the air* to body temperature.

- The respiratory system is divided into upper and lower respiratory systems. The *upper respiratory system* includes the nasal and oral cavities, paranasal sinuses, pharynx, and larynx.

- The *lower respiratory system* includes the trachea, bronchial ducts, and lungs.

THE UPPER RESPIRATORY SYSTEM

Nasal Cavity

- The *nasal cavity* is a hollow space behind the nose and is divided by the *nasal septum*. The *nasal conchae* with their curved surfaces and moist mucous membranes swirl and warm air as it enters the nasal cavity.

- The mucus secreted by the mucous membrane mixes with the air and filters out particles, preventing them from entering the respiratory system. Blood vessels are found on the surface of the nasal conchae and aid in the warming of inhaled air.

- Tiny hairlike structures or *cilia* arise from the mucous membrane in the nasal cavity. As the air passes over these structures, they enhance the process of trapping particles, preventing them from entering the respiratory tract.

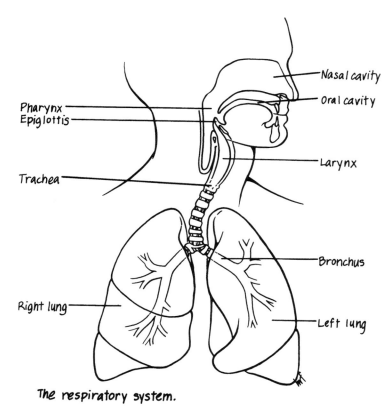

The respiratory system.

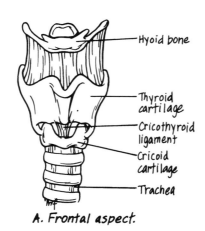

A. Frontal aspect.

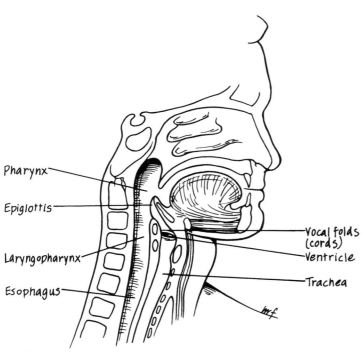

B. Lateral aspect.
Frontal and lateral aspects of larynx.

Oral Cavity

- The *oral cavity*, described in Chapter 9, is the opening to the alimentary canal that serves as a passageway for food and air. Cleaning and filtering mechanisms, such as the surface blood vessels, conchae, and cilia present in the nasal cavity, are absent from the oral cavity.

Paranasal Sinuses

- The *paranasal sinuses,* described in Chapter 4, are air-filled cavities located within bones of the skull. They include the *frontal, ethmoid, sphenoid,* and *maxillary sinuses.*

- Each pair of sinuses empties into the nasal cavity for drainage and acts as a passageway for air.

- The sinuses function to provide *resonance for speech* and serve to *lighten the weight of the skull.*

Pharynx

- The *pharynx* serves as part of the gastro-intestinal tract during the passage of food and as part of the respiratory system during the passage of air.

Larynx

- The *larynx,* also known as the *voice box,* separates the pharynx from the trachea. It serves as a passageway for air and helps change sound into words for speech.

- The larynx has a flap that prevents food particles from entering the trachea.

- The shape of the larynx is maintained by cartilage, with the *thyroid cartilage* and the *hyoid bone* covering the anterior wall. The posterior wall is supported by *cricoid arytenoid* and *corniculate cartilages.*

- On the upper surface is the *epiglottic cartilage,* which has a flap extending upward called the *epiglottis.* During the passage of air the flap remains up and air enters the larynx. When swallowing occurs, pressure on the epiglottis from the food bolus causes the flap to close the opening to the larynx, preventing food from entering the larynx and trachea.

Trachea

- The *trachea* or *windpipe* is located between the larynx and the primary bronchus in front of the esophagus and behind the sternum. The trachea serves as a *passageway for air* entering the bronchial tree.

- The trachea is round, with rings containing cartilage which supports and keeps the trachea open. The inner lining of the trachea is a mucous membrane with ciliated or hairlike structures which continue to cleanse the air as it passes through. The mucus secreted by the mucous membrane continues to filter the air before it enters the lungs.

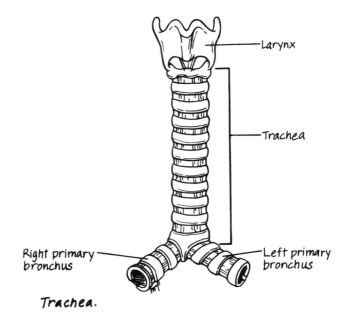

Trachea.

Bronchial Ducts

- The trachea branches at its distal end (the level of the fifth thoracic vertebra) to become the right primary bronchus and the left primary bronchus. The right and left primary bronchi are the main air passageways to the lungs.

- The thoracic cavity contains the *mediastinal structures*, including the heart which rests more on the left side. The primary bronchus and the size of the lobes of the lungs vary to accommodate the mediastinal structures.

- The *right primary bronchus* is wider and more vertical than the left bronchus and therefore is susceptible to foreign objects entering its passageway. The *left primary bronchus* is smaller in diameter and turns more horizontally.

- The primary bronchi branch to form a tree structure usually referred to as the *bronchial tree*. The first branching forms the *secondary bronchi*, which again branch and become smaller *tertiary bronchi* and *bronchioles*. The bronchial tree terminates at the tiny *terminal bronchioles*, which connect with *alveolar ducts* and finally with alveoli. Most of the bronchial tree contains cartilage which provides support to keep the passageway open.

- *Alveoli* are small, grapelike clusters or "air sacs" which are surrounded by a network of capillaries. The membrane of the alveoli is very thin, facilitating the transfer of oxygen and carbon dioxide during respiration.

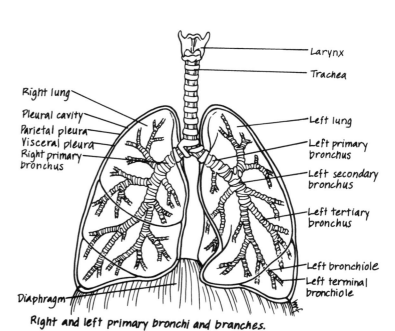

Right and left primary bronchi and branches.

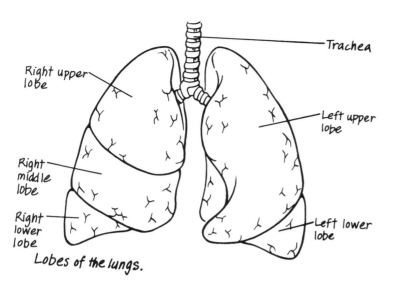

Lobes of the lungs.

Lungs

- The *lungs* resemble two cone-shaped structures located on each side of the mediastinum. They have a spongelike structure, which provides support for the bronchial tree and alveoli, and they are covered by the *pleural membrane*. The *parietal pleura* lines the interior walls of the thoracic cavity, and the *visceral pleura* covers the surface of the lungs.

- Located between the parietal and visceral pleurae is the *pleural cavity*, which is filled with fluid that lubricates the coverings of the wall and lungs, thus preventing friction as the lungs expand against the ribs during respiration.

- The right lung is larger than the left lung and is divided into three lobes called the *right upper lobe, right middle lobe,* and *right lower lobe.* The smaller left lung has only two lobes, the *left upper lobe* and the *left lower lobe.*

Respiration and Air Exchange

- The process of respiration is facilitated by atmospheric pressure and regulated by the special breathing center located in the brainstem.

- The air pressure inside the tiny alveoli and the air pressure outside the thoracic cavity remain nearly the same. If the air pressure inside the alveoli drops, air will be taken in from the outside to maintain air pressure. The *rate of respiration* is controlled by the *brainstem*, and the *need for oxygen* by the *cells*.

- During breathing or inhalation, the diaphragm lowers and the lungs expand, sucking in air to fill the alveoli. As air is released or exhaled, the diaphragm relaxes, returning to its normal position, and the lungs return to their more normal size. During relaxation, a residual amount of air remains in the lungs.

- The walls of the alveoli are semipermeable, permitting oxygen to move across the membrane to oxygenate blood by the process of diffusion. Simultaneously, carbon dioxide to be exhaled diffuses across the membrane from the blood.

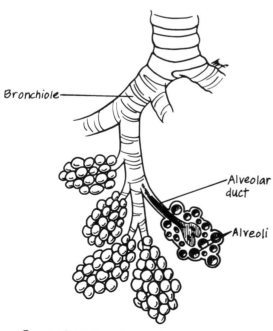

Bronchiole terminates in alveolar duct with alveoli clusters surrounding ducts. Capillary structures surround the alveoli permitting exchange of oxygen and carbon dioxide.

- During breathing about 500 ml of air (tidal volume) is moved in and out of the lungs. The amount of residual air that remains in the lungs at all times is about 1200 ml.

- In disorders such as *emphysema*, the lungs loose their elasticity and air becomes trapped in the alveoli. The walls of the alveoli harden, preventing the exchange of air from taking place.

PATHOPHYSIOLOGIC TERMS ASSOCIATED WITH THE RESPIRATORY SYSTEM

Adenocystic carcinoma a malignancy associated with the mucous glands of the respiratory tract

Allergic rhinitis an allergic response by the nasal mucosa

Alveolar cell carcinoma a malignancy that originates in the bronchioles and later spreads to the alveoli

Apnea the absence of breathing

Atelectasis a partial or complete collapse of a lung

Bronchial adenoma slow-growing tumor of the bronchial mucous membranes

Bronchiectasis chronic dilation of the bronchus or bronchioles

Bronchitis inflammation of the lining of the bronchus

Bronchogenic carcinoma a malignancy originating in the primary bronchi

Bronchopneumonia an inflammation of the lungs originating in the bronchioles

Bronchospasm a spasm of the muscular tissue of the bronchi

Cheyne-Stokes respiration repeated cycles of irregular breathing

Dyspnea difficulty in breathing

Emphysema a chronic lung disease characterized by increased size of alveoli and destruction of the walls causing trapping of air in the lungs

Hemothorax the presence of blood in the pleural cavity

Hyperventilation prolonged rapid deep breathing

Influenza a contagious respiratory disease transmitted by airborne microorganisms

Laryngitis an inflammation of the larynx

Legionnaires' disease an acute form of bacterial pneumonia

Pleurisy an inflammation of the pleura

Pneumoconiosis a chronic condition caused by inhalation of material such as asbestos or dust particles

Pneumonia inflammation and congestion in the lungs

Pneumothorax the presence of air in the pleural cavity

Pulmonary edema an accumulation of fluid in the lungs

Pulmonary fibrosis a progressive disease characterized by the formation of fibrous tissues in the walls of the alveoli

Rhinitis an inflammation of the nasal mucosa

Tuberculosis an infectious disease caused by the *Mycobacterium tuberculosis* organism.

Chapter 12 Practice Questions

1. **The parts of the upper respiratory system include the**
   a. nasal cavity, oral cavity, pharynx, and trachea.
   b. oral cavity, paranasal sinuses, trachea, and larynx.
   c. trachea, bronchial tree, lungs, and alveoli.
   d. nasal cavity, pharynx, paranasal sinuses, and larynx.

2. **Structure or mechanisms that filter, cleanse, and warm the air before it enters the lungs include all of the following except**
   a. cilia.
   b. mucus.
   c. epiglottis.
   d. nasal conchae.

3. **The organ of the respiratory system that serves as a passageway for air and changes sound into speech is the**
   a. oral cavity.
   b. larynx.
   c. trachea.
   d. primary bronchus.

4. **The _____ bronchus is smaller in diameter and turns more horizontally.**
   a. right primary
   b. left primary
   c. right secondary
   d. left secondary

5. **The membrane covering the lungs is the**
   a. alveolus.
   b. parietal pleura.
   c. visceral pleura.
   d. pleurisy.

6. The rate of respiration is controlled by the
   a. brainstem.
   b. cerebrum.
   c. lungs.
   d. larynx.

7. The amount of air moved in and out of the lungs during normal breathing is called the
   a. respiration volume.
   b. tidal volume.
   c. residual volume.
   d. exchange volume.

8. The chronic lung disease that traps air in the lung as a result of destruction of the walls of the alveoli is
   a. adenocystic carcinoma.
   b. alveolar cell carcinoma.
   c. atelectasis.
   d. emphysema.

9. An inflammation of the membrane covering the lungs is called
   a. pleurisy.
   b. pneumonia.
   c. pneumoconiosis.
   d. pulmonary edema.

10. An inflammation of the nasal cavity due to allergies is referred to as
    a. apnea.
    b. dyspnea.
    c. rhinitis.
    d. allergic rhinitis.

The Urinary System

THE URINARY SYSTEM

- The *urinary system* functions to *remove waste materials* from the blood that would become toxic to the body if not eliminated. In addition, this system plays an important role in the *formation of red blood cells* and in *maintenance of the water and electrolyte balance* and the *pH level of body fluids*.

- The organs of the urinary system are the *kidneys, ureters, urinary bladder,* and *urethra*.

KIDNEY

- The kidneys are bean-shaped structures located in the *retroperitoneal space* on each side of the vertebral column. Each kidney is enclosed by a membrane called a *renal capsule*.

- The kidneys are located at the level from the twelfth thoracic vertebra to the third lumbar vertebra. The left kidney is located slightly higher (by 1 to 2 cm) than the right kidney. During respiration the kidneys drop slightly as the diaphragm is lowered. When the body is in the erect position, the kidneys fall lower in the abdominal cavity.

- The *hilum* is situated on a concave surface on the medial aspect of the kidney. Major vessels including the ureters, renal arteries, and veins and lymphatic vessels enter and exit the kidney through the hilar area.

- The *renal artery*, which branches from the abdominal aorta, provides the blood supply to the kidney, and the *renal vein* drains blood from the kidney to the inferior vena cava.

- The *ureters* empty urine from the kidney at the hilum.

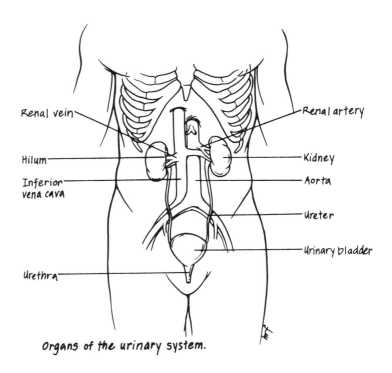

Organs of the urinary system.

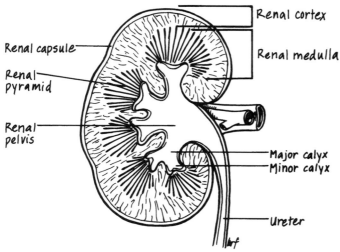

Cross-section showing internal structure of the kidney.

- The main body of the kidney has two major sections: the *renal cortex* located more on the outer surface of the kidney, and the *renal medulla* located in the midsection of the kidney.

- The outer renal cortex has a granular appearance because of the arrangement of numerous tiny functional units of the kidney called *nephrons*. Tissue from the cortex drops into the medullary tissue, producing a striated appearance in the tissue.

- The *medulla* is the inner portion of the kidney made up mainly of *renal pyramids*.

- The kidney plays an important role in the production of red blood cells. As the level of hemoglobin drops, the kidneys produce *erythropoietin*, a hormone that stimulates the red bone marrow to produce more red blood cells.

The Nephron Unit

- There are approximately 1 million nephron units in a kidney. A nephron unit is a tiny, winding tubule surrounded by a vast network of blood vessels; it originates in the cortex and has loops that dip into the medulla. This unit is the *functional unit* of the kidney where blood is filtered and urine is formed. In addition, the nephron filters substances from the blood, producing a filtrate, and then reclaims some of the same substances from the filtrate and returns them to the blood before it leaves the nephron unit.

- At the origin of the nephron unit is the *renal corpuscle*, a small sac containing the *glomerulus* which has an extremely thin wall encircled by *Bowman's capsule*. Bowman's capsule is at the beginning of the renal tubule which travels a winding path through the nephron unit. The portion of the tubule nearest Bowman's capsule is called the *proximal convoluted tubule*.

- The proximal convoluted tubule dips, producing an uncoiled section called the *loop of Henle*. The loop of Henle turns, producing one long loop, and the tubule begins another winding path called the *distal convoluted tubule*.

Nephron unit.

- The distal convoluted tubule opens into a large collecting duct within the medulla. In the medulla the tubule opens into a larger collecting vessel called the *minor calyx*, which empties into the *major calyx*.

- The major calyx opens into the large funnel-shaped *renal pelvis*, which narrows as it exits the hilum to become the ureter.

Blood Circulation to and from the Nephron Unit

- Blood vessels surround the renal corpuscle and renal tubule. Blood reaches the kidney via the *renal artery* which branches into *interlobar arteries*. The blood vessels from the interlobar arteries continue to branch into smaller vessels called *arciform* and *interlobular arteries*.

- The interlobular artery branches into the *afferent arteriole,* which delivers blood directly to the renal capsule and the glomerulus. As the blood moves through the glomerulus, its is filtered, and the filtrate moves into Bowman's capsule and into the renal tubule. The blood leaves the renal capsule by the *efferent arteriole* and enters the *capillary network* surrounding the proximal convoluted tubule, loop of Henle, and distal convoluted tubule. As the blood travels through the network surrounding the renal tubule, dissolved substances are reclaimed by the blood. From this capillary network blood returns through a corresponding venous system to the renal vein and vena cava.

URETERS

- The *ureters* connect the kidneys to the urinary bladder. Their origin is in the renal pelvis at the hilum, and they drop behind the peritoneum to the posterior inferior surface of the urinary bladder. They are approximately 25 cm in length and lie on each side of the vertebral column.

- The ureters open into the interior of the urinary bladder through flaps which prevent backflow of urine from the bladder to the ureters.

- The walls of the ureters include muscular tissue which provides peristalsis for movement of urine through the ureters.

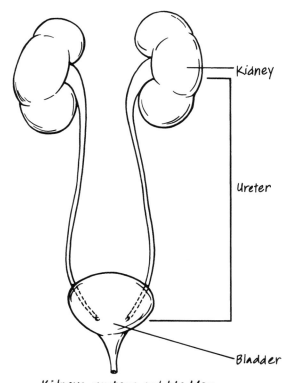

Kidneys, ureters and bladder.

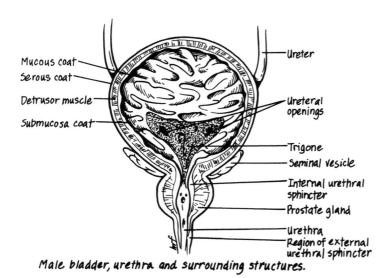

Male bladder, urethra and surrounding structures.

Mucous coat
Serous coat
Detrusor muscle
Submucosa coat

Ureter
Ureteral openings
Trigone
Seminal vesicle
Internal urethral sphincter
Prostate gland
Urethra
Region of external urethral sphincter

URINARY BLADDER

- The *urinary bladder* is a hollow muscular structure serving as a *reservoir* for holding urine. When it is empty, the walls form folds over one another. As urine fills the bladder, the walls begin to expand and retain the urine until the need for elimination. A normal urinary bladder can hold a maximum of 700 ml. When the capacity reaches about 300 to 400 ml, receptors in the walls of the bladder are stimulated, creating a desire to eliminate the urine (urination).

- Near the middle of the floor of the bladder is the *trigone,* an area shaped like a triangle. The *apex* of the trigone is the opening to the urethra, and the two *base points* of the trigone are the openings connecting to the ureters.

- The inner layer of tissue in the urinary bladder consists of mucous membrane and is layered with multiple layers of epithelial cells. The outer layer is the muscular layer and includes the *detrusor* and *internal urethral sphincter* muscles. Sustained contraction of the urethral sphincter muscle prevents urine from leaving the bladder.

URETHRA

- The *urethra* is the tube or passageway for eliminating urine from the bladder to the outside of the body. The urethra muscular structure includes the *external urethral sphincter* muscle.

- Urination involves relaxation of the external urethral sphincter and contraction of the detrusor muscle in the urinary bladder walls.

FORMATION OF URINE

- The process of urine formation begins in the renal capsule as blood enters the glomerulus. The pressure within the glomerular capillaries facilitates the filtering of substances from the blood through the glomerular membranes. Water and other dissolved substances are removed from the blood by this process, forming the *filtrate.*

- The rate of filtration is directly related to the pressure within the glomerular capillaries. For an average adult the rate of filtrate production is approximately 125 ml/min or 180 L/day.

- The *glomerular filtrate* is received by Bowman's capsule and moved into the renal tubule.

- The filtrate travels through the proximal convoluted tubule, the loop of Henle, and the distal convoluted tubule. As it passes through the tubule, water is reabsorbed by the blood. Other materials are also reabsorbed by the blood, including glucose, amino acids, sodium, potassium, and calcium. This process of reabsorption allows the kidneys to maintain the water and electrolyte balance in the body.

- The amount of filtrate significantly decreases as it passes through the renal tubule as a result of reabsorption processes by which water and other substances are returned to the blood plasma. The total amount of urine eliminated during a 24-hour period is from 0.5 to 2.5 L.

- The presence of certain substances or an increase in their amount in the urine may be a symptom of a disease or disorder. For example, the presence of *glucose* in urine (glycosuria) may be a symptom of a disorder associated with glucose metabolism such as type I diabetes mellitus.

- *Urea* may be present in urine in a limited amount. Urea is a by-product of protein metabolism found in the glomerular filtrate but is only partially absorbed, the remainder being excreted in urine.

- *Uric acid* is also a by-product of protein metabolism; about 90 percent of it is reabsorbed by the nephron unit, and the other 10 percent is eliminated in the urine.

PATHOPHYSIOLOGIC TERMINOLOGY ASSOCIATED WITH THE URINARY SYSTEM

Anuria a lack of urine

Cystitis an inflammation of the urinary bladder usually caused by bacterial infection or mechanical injury

Cystocele herniation of the urinary bladder through the vaginal wall

Dysuria painful urination

Glomerulonephritis an inflammation in the glomerulus

Hematuria the presence of red blood cells in the urine

Hydronephrosis enlargement or distension of the kidney due to an obstructed ureter

Hypercalciuri an excessive amount of calcium in the urine

Incontinence the inability to control urination

Nephritis an inflammation in the kidney

Nephromegaly an enlarged kidney

Nephroptosis the condition in which a kidney has dropped from its normal position

Polycystic disease an inherited disorder in which multiple cysts are present along the nephron unit

Polyuria excessive urination

Pyelitis an inflammation of the renal pelvis

Pyelonephritis an inflammation of the kidney due to an infection

Renal calculi or kidney stones solidified salts forming stones found in the urinary tract; may be located in the kidney, ureters, or urinary bladder; can cause pain and bleeding and obstruct the drainage system of the kidney

Renal cell carcinoma a malignant tumor of the kidney which usually metastasizes

Renal colic the presence of pain caused by the passage of a stone or calculus in the kidney or ureter

Transitional cell carcinoma a malignancy usually affecting the urinary bladder

Uremia the condition in which toxic metabolic waste products are not removed from the blood because of renal dysfunction

Urinary tract infection (UTI) the presence of microorganisms in the urine, indicating that an infection may be present somewhere in the urinary system.

Chapter 13 Practice Questions

1. **The kidneys are covered by a membrane called the**
   a. renal peritoneum.
   b. hilum.
   c. renal capsule.
   d. renal hilar membrane.

2. **Blood, lymphatic vessels, and nerves enter the kidney through the**
   a. retroperitoneal space.
   b. hilar area.
   c. major calyx.
   d. minor calyx.

3. **The blood supply to the kidney is through the**
   a. renal artery.
   b. renal vein.
   c. ureters.
   d. medulla.

4. **The nephron unit is located in the**
   a. medulla of the kidney.
   b. cortex of the tissue.
   c. renal corpuscle.
   d. renal tubule.

5. **Blood is filtered in**
   a. the glomerulus.
   b. Bowman's capsule.
   c. the renal tubule.
   d. the loop of Henle.

6. **The proximal and distal convoluted tubules are part of the**
   a. calyces.
   b. pyramids.
   c. nephron unit.
   d. afferent artery drainage system.

7. **Blood enters the renal corpuscle by the**
   a. afferent arteries.
   b. efferent arteries.
   c. interlobar arteries.
   d. interlobular arteries.

8. **Urine enters the urinary bladder posteriorly and inferiorly at the**
   a. apex of the trigone.
   b. base of the trigone.
   c. detrusor sphincter.
   d. internal sphincter muscle.

9. **An inherited disorder of the kidney characterized by multiple cysts along the nephron unit is called**
   a. glomerulonephritis.
   b. nephritis.
   c. nephroptosis.
   d. polycystic disease.

10. **An inflammation in the kidney is called**
    a. cystitis.
    b. nephritis.
    c. hydronephrosis.
    d. uremia.

The Female and Male Reproductive Systems

- The organs of the *reproductive system* are designed primarily to provide continuation of the human species. If organs of the reproductive system are removed, such as the ovaries, uterus, breast, or testes, the survival of the individual is not affected.

- The *primary sex organs* are called gonads. *Gonads* produce sex cells, and, when they are fertilized, an offspring is produced based on DNA information from both sex cells (egg and sperm).

- The organs of the female and male reproductive systems differ in structure and function. Both sexes secrete hormones that support and protect the production and fertilization of sex cells to ensure survival of the species.

FEMALE REPRODUCTIVE SYSTEM

- The *female reproductive system* is designed to produce sex cells (egg cells) and, after fertilization, to nourish and support the development of the egg cell into an *embryo* and then into a *fetus*. The uterus holds the fetus during the development period before birth. The *mammary glands* support the development of milk to nourish the newborn after birth.

- The primary sex organ in females is the *ovary*. Other organs located both internally and externally serve as accessory organs.

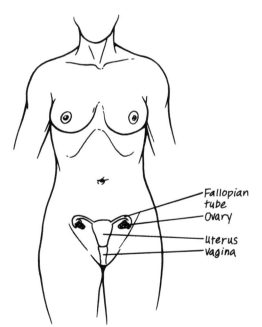

Female reproductive organs (ovaries located in abdominal cavity).

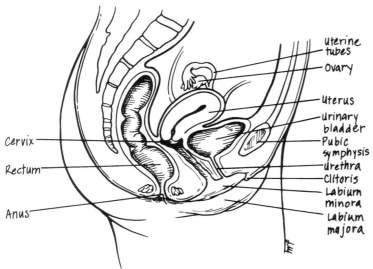

Lateral aspect of female reproductive and accessory organs.

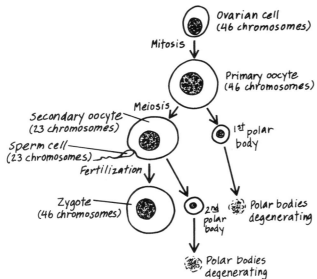

Oogenesis. If fertilization occurs the secondary oocyte divides to become a small second polar and a large zygote.

- The internal accessory organs include the *uterus, fallopian (uterine) tubes,* and *vagina.* The external organs (vulva) *are the labia majora, labia minora, clitoris, and Bartholin's glands.*

- The mammary glands in the breast are also considered accessory organs of the female reproductive system.

Ovaries

- The *ovaries* have an oval shape and are located in the pelvic cavity, one on each side of the midsagittal plane. Each ovary has a medulla and a cortex.

- The *medulla* is the supporting connective, blood, nervous, and lymphatic tissue.

- The *outer cortex* holds the follicle covered by a thin epithelial layer called the *germinal epithelium.* The follicle is the site of egg cell development.

- Before a female is born, millions of *primordial follicles* are formed in the cortex. Each follicle has one large cell called a *primary oocyte* and several follicle cells.

- Early in development, the primary oocyte begins *meiosis* (sex cell division) and then ceases, remaining in this state until puberty.

- At puberty, follicle stimulating hormone (FSH) is secreted by the pituitary gland, and follicle maturation occurs. The oocyte begins meiosis, producing a daughter cell having only one-half the number of chromosomes as the parent cell. This process leads to the production of an egg cell (ovum) which when fertilized by a sperm cell from the male results in an embryo.

- *Ovulation* is the process by which a primary oocyte undergoes *oogenesis,* producing a *secondary oocyte* and a *first polar body.* The oocyte is then released by the ovary. The *fallopian tube* is designed to receive the egg cell and conduct it through to the uterus. If the egg cell is not fertilized within a short period of time, it begins to degenerate and is eventually eliminated.

- At the time of ovulation, the follicle from which the egg originates grows larger and is filled with fluid, becoming the *corpus luteum*. The corpus luteum secretes hormones, and if the egg is fertilized, it will continue to do so. If no fertilization occurs, the hormone secretions from the corpus luteum diminish, eventually ceasing all together.

Fallopian Tubes

- The *fallopian tubes* have funnel-shaped openings or *infundibula* near the ovary which are designed to receive the oocyte. The secretions from the inner walls of the fallopian tubes enhance the ability of the oocyte to enter the tube. Once it has entered, the egg cell moves toward the uterus.

Uterus

- The *uterus* is an upside-down pear-shaped organ with multiple functions. It has the ability to sustain development of the embryo and fetus. It also holds and protects the egg cell as it waits to be fertilized.

- The corpus luteum, resulting from ovulation, secretes progesterone which stimulates the wall of the uterus. If the egg is fertilized, the wall of the uterus will sustain the embryo for development. If the egg is not fertilized, the corpus luteum will stop producing progesterone and the uterine walls will slough away, producing menstrual flow.

- The inner walls of the uterus are lined with *endometrium*. The middle layer is known as the *myometrium*, a muscular layer. Both these layers undergo tremendous change during pregnancy when they are stretched to hold the fetus and eventually contract to expel the newborn.

- The outer covering of the uterus is called the *perimetrium*.

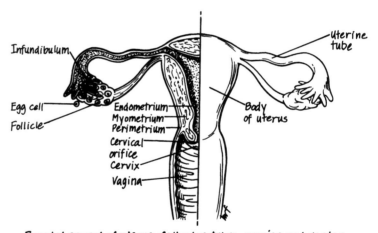

Frontal aspect of uterus, fallopian tubes, ovaries and vagina.

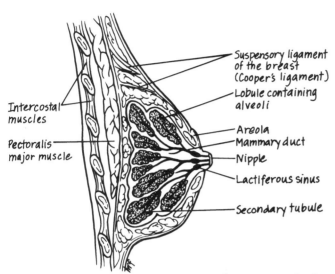

Breast tissue showing structure of mammary glands.

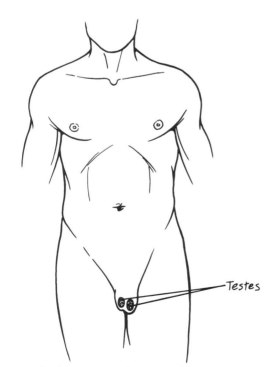

Testes located in scrotum.

Accessory Organs

- The *vagina* is a muscular tube connecting the uterus to the outside of the body. It lies posterior to the bladder and anterior to the rectum. During the birth process the vagina must stretch to accommodate the passage of the baby. Located on either side of the opening of the vagina are *Bartholin glands* which produce a lubricant.

- The *labia majora* enclose and protect the external reproductive glands and lie close together separated by a long opening to cover the urethral and vaginal openings.

- The *labia minora* are folds located within the cleft covered by the labia majora.

- The *clitoris* is a small projection near the end of the vulva and corresponds to the male penis in that erectile tissue is present.

- *Mammary glands* are located in the breast and function to secrete milk during pregnancy.

- Development of the mammary glands is controlled by hormones secreted by the ovaries.

- *Breast tissue* is composed of adipose and connective tissue consisting of lobules and multiple ducts with milk-secreting cells. The ducts lead to the nipple where milk is secreted.

- The *nipple* is the tip of each breast; it is surrounded by pigmented skin called the *areola*.

- Male and female mammary glands are similar, however, only the female glands continue to develop at puberty.

MALE REPRODUCTIVE SYSTEM

- The *primary sex organ* of the male is the *testes*, where sperm cells are formed. Accessory glands are present for support, protection, and movement of the sex cells.

- The interior accessory organs are the *epididymis, vas deferens, ejaculatory ducts, urethra, seminal vesicles, prostate gland,* and *bulbourethral glands.*

- The external accessory organs are the scrotum and penis.

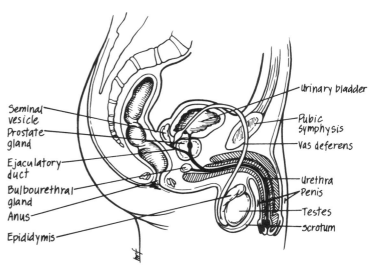

Male reproductive and accessory organs.

Testes

- The *testes* are found within a fibrous capsule located inside the scrotum and have a structure consisting of multiple lobules.

- Each lobule contains *seminiferous tubules* which are coiled and would reach to about 70 cm if straightened out. These tubules form a network that becomes a tube called the *epididymis.*

- The seminiferous tubules are lined with germinal epithelium which produces male sex cells called sperm. The production of sperm cells continues to occur throughout the reproductive life of the male.

- As the sperm are produced through a process called *spermatogenesis,* they pass through to the epididymis where they undergo maturation.

- The sperm cell has a large head, compared to the rest of the cell, and a long, thin tail. The nucleus is located in the head of the sperm along with the chromosomes. The head also contains an enzyme that facilitates penetration of the membrane of the egg cell.

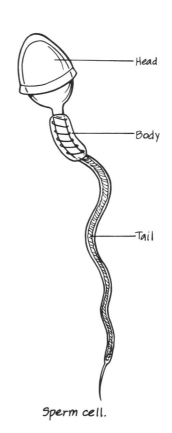

Sperm cell.

Accessory Organs

- The *epididymis* is a tubule with multiple coils connecting the testes to the vas deferens. After the sperm move into the epididymis they remain there for a period of time to complete maturation.

- The *vas deferens* is a tube passing from the medial side of the testes into the abdominal cavity and ending posterior to the urinary bladder. An alkaline fluid is secreted by the lining of the vas deferens, which helps maintain the correct pH environment for the sperm cells.

- The *prostate gland* is a bulb-shaped gland surrounding the urethra just below the bladder. This gland has ducts opening into the urethra. Secretions from the prostate gland help maintain the correct pH environment and support sperm cell motility.

- The *bulbourethral glands* are about the size of peas and are located inferior to the prostate gland where they are enclosed by the external urethral sphincter. These glands secrete a mucuslike fluid in response to sexual stimulation. *Seminal fluid* from the bulbourethral glands and sperm cells is expelled through the urethra during sexual stimulation.

- The *scrotum* is a sac that covers the testes, supporting smooth movement of these organs and helping to maintain the proper temperature for the production of sperm cells.

- The *penis* is a cylindrical organ which becomes the passageway through which urine and seminal fluid are expelled. The walls of the penis contain muscular erectile tissue which facilitates erection of the penis during sexual intercourse, as well as the passage of sperm cells into the vagina and into the egg cell in the female.

PATHOPHYSIOLOGIC TERMINOLOGY ASSOCIATED WITH THE FEMALE AND MALE REPRODUCTIVE SYSTEMS

Amenorrhea the absence of menstrual flow

Breast cancer the most common cancer found in women; can be one of a variety of types

Cervical cancer a malignancy of the cervix of the uterus; can be detected early through a Pap smear.

Prostate cancer the second leading cause of cancer deaths in men; characterized by painful and difficult urination; if found and treated early, a long survival period will result

Testicular cancer a malignancy occurring usually between the ages of 15 and 34 in males; treatment involves removal of the diseased testis

Dysmenorrhea painful menstrual flow

Endometritis an inflammation of the endometrium

Epididymitis an inflammation of the epididymis

Gonorrhea a sexually transmitted disease producing infection of genital mucous membranes

Gynecomastia an abnormal enlargement of the male breast

Herpes genitalis an infection caused by herpesvirus

Oophoritis an inflammation of an ovary

Prolapsed uterus protruson of the uterus into the vaginal opening

Prostatitis an inflammation of the prostate gland

Salpingitis an inflammation of the fallopian tube or tubes

Syphilis an acute, contagious infection characterized by sores as the first symptom; can spread to other organs in the body

Trichomoniasis an inflammation of the mucous membrane of the vagina producing a yellowish discharge

Vaginitis an inflammation of the vagina

Chapter 14 Practice Questions

1. **The primary sex organ in females is the**

   a. mammary gland.
   b. ovary.
   c. uterus.
   d. cervix.

2. **The primary sex organ in males is the**

   a. vas deferens.
   b. epididymis.
   c. scrotum.
   d. testes.

3. **Division of sex cells is called**

   a. mitosis.
   b. meiosis.
   c. oogenesis.
   d. the corpus luteum.

4. **The organ that hold the embryo and fetus during development is the**

   a. ovary.
   b. fallopian tube.
   c. uterus.
   d. vagina.

5. **An inflammation of the inner lining of the uterus is called**
   a. endometritis.
   b. oophoritis.
   c. amenorrhea.
   d. epididymitis.

Bibliography

Austrin MG, Austrin HR. *Learning Medical Terminology,* 8th ed. Mosby Lifeline, St. Louis, 1995.

Ballinger PW. *Merrill's Atlas of Radiographic Positions and Radiologic Procedures,* Vols. I-III, 7th ed. Mosby-Year Book, St. Louis, 1991.

Hole JW Jr. *Essentials of Human Anatomy and Physiology,* 3rd ed. WC Brown, Dubuque, Iowa, 1989.

Laudicina PF. *Applied Pathology for Radiographers.* WB Saunders, Philadelphia, 1989.

Möller T, Reif E, Stark P. *Pocket Atlas of Radiographic Anatomy.* Thieme, Stuttgart, 1993.

O'Toole M, ed. *Encyclopedia and Dictionary of Medicine, Nursing, and Allied Health,* 5th ed. WB Saunders, Philadelphia, 1992.

Tortora G. *Principles of Human Anatomy.* HarperCollins, New York, 1992.

Answers

Chapter 1
1. d
2. b
3. c
4. b
5. a
6. c
7. d
8. a
9. c
10. a
11. c
12. a
13. d
14. c
15. b

Chapter 2
1. c
2. b
3. a
4. d
5. a
6. b
7. d
8. b
9. a
10. b

Chapter 3
1. a
2. c
3. d
4. d
5. c
6. c
7. b
8. a
9. d
10. d
11. a
12. d
13. b
14. d

15. d
16. b
17. a
18. d
19. a
20. b
21. a
22. c
23. d
24. c
25. b

Chapter 4
1. b
2. d
3. d
4. c
5. d
6. a
7. a
8. b
9. d
10. c
11. a
12. d
13. b
14. c
15. d
16. c
17. a
18. c
19. c
20. d
21. c
22. b
23. c
24. d
25. b

Chapter 5
1. a
2. d
3. b
4. c

5. b
6. a
7. c
8. b
9. b
10. b
11. c
12. a

Chapter 6
1. a
2. c
3. c
4. d
5. c
6. d
7. d
8. a
9. a
10. d

Chapter 7
1. b
2. d
3. b
4. c
5. b
6. d
7. c
8. b
9. d
10. a

Chapter 8
1. c
2. a
3. d
4. c
5. d
6. c
7. b
8. d
9. c
10. b

Chapter 9
1. c
2. b
3. a
4. c
5. c
6. b
7. a
8. a
9. b
10. d

Chapter 10
1. a
2. c
3. d
4. a
5. c
6. a
7. a
8. c
9. b
10. c

Chapter 11
1. a
2. c
3. d
4. d
5. b

Chapter 12
1. d
2. c
3. b
4. b
5. c
6. a
7. b
8. d
9. a
10. d

Chapter 13
1. c
2. b
3. a
4. b
5. a

6. c
7. a
8. b
9. d
10. b

Chapter 14
1. b
2. d
3. b
4. c
5. a

ISBN 0-07-009231-1

90000

9 780070 092310

BURNS: ANATOMY &
PHYSIOLOGY